Clinical Optics

Other books of interest

Clinical Orthoptics
Fiona Rowe
0 632 04274 5

Diagnosis and Management of Ocular Mobility Disorders
Second Edition
A. Anson & H. Davis
0 632 04798 4

Ocular Anatomy and Physiology
T. Saude
0 632 03599 4

Clinical Anatomy of the Eye
R.S. Snell & M.A. Lemp
0 632 04344 X

Orthoptic Assessment and Management
Second Edition
D. Stidwill
0 632 05012 8

Clinical Optics

Third Edition

Andrew R. Elkington

CBE, MA, FRCS, FRCOphth
Consultant Ophthalmologist
Southampton Eye Unit
Southampton General Hospital.
Professor of Ophthalmology
University of Southampton.
President, Royal College of
Ophthalmologists
(1994–1997).

Helena J. Frank

BMedSci, FRCS, FRCOphth
Consultant Ophthalmologist
Royal Victoria Hospital
Bournemouth.

Michael J. Greaney

MD, FRCSEd, FRCOphth
Specialist Registrar
Southampton Eye Unit
Southampton General Hospital.

Blackwell
Science

Editorial offices:
Blackwell Science Ltd, 9600 Garsington Road, Oxford OX4 2DQ, UK
    Tel: +44 (0) 1865 776868
Blackwell Publishing Inc., 350 Main Street, Malden, MA 02148-5020, USA
    Tel: +1 781 388 8250
Blackwell Science Asia Pty Ltd, 550 Swanston Street, Carlton, Victoria 3053, Australia
    Tel: +61 (0)3 8359 1011

First edition published 1984
Reprinted 1988
Second edition published 1991
Reprinted 1995, 1997
Third edition published 1999
Reprinted 2002, 2004, 2005, 2006

ISBN-10: 0-632-04989-8
ISBN-13: 978-0-632-04989-9

Library of Congress Cataloging-in-Publication Data
Elkington, A.R.
        Clinical optics / Andrew R. Elkington, Helena
J. Frank, Michael J. Greaney.–3rd ed.
        p. cm.
        Includes bibliographical references and
index.
        ISBN 0-632-04989-8 (pbk.)
        1. Physiological optics. 2. Optics. I. Frank,
Helena J. II. Greaney, Michael J. III. Title.
        [DNLM: 1. Eye Diseases–physiopathology.
2. Lenses. 3. Optics. 4. Refraction, Ocular
WW 300 E43c 1999]
QP475.E48 1999
617.7'5–dc21
DNLM/DLC
for Library of Congress   99-20296
                                                        CIP

A catalogue record for this title is available from the British Library

Set in 10/13 pt Palatino
by DP Photosetting, Aylesbury, Bucks

The publisher's policy is to use permanent paper from mills that operate a sustainable forestry policy, and which has been manufactured from pulp processed using acid-free and elementary chlorine-free practices. Furthermore, the publisher ensures that the text paper and cover board used have met acceptable environmental accreditation standards.

For further information on Blackwell Publishing, visit our website:
www.blackwellpublishing.com

Contents

Preface to the Third Edition

In the preface to the second edition of this book we stressed that we had written the text in the hope of helping those trainee eye surgeons who were preparing to take their basic professional examinations. We assumed that the optics they had learned at school had long since been forgotten, and we therefore set out to explain the subject from first principles.

Our aim was to keep the text logical and simple and we used diagrams liberally to complement the written word. These diagrams themselves were simplified so that they could be both easily memorised and reproduced – even under the stress of examination conditions.

Throughout the book we emphasised the clinical relevance of each topic and we hoped that this approach would allow readers to understand better the optical problems experienced by many of their patients.

During the eight years since that edition was published, many changes have taken place in the practice of ophthalmology. New methods of examination have become available, including sophisticated automated visual field analysers. There have been great advances in the design of intraocular lenses. Corneal refractive surgery has become more popular and also more complex. There are many new types of lasers in clinical use. All these advances depend upon the application of basic optical concepts in new settings.

In writing this third edition we have taken the opportunity to identify these principles and to explain their application in the context of modern ophthalmic practice. In so doing our aim remains the same, namely to enhance the care of patients by helping ophthalmologists to master the optical principles that underpin so much of their everyday work.

Acknowledgements

It is a pleasure to pay a tribute to Dr. Jock Anderson OBE FRCS, who both commented on the typescript and prepared the index.

We thank, too, our Publishers for inviting us to write the third edition and for their subsequent encouragement and support in the preparation of this book.

A.R.E.
H.J.F.
M.J.G.
April 1999

1 Properties of Light and Visual Function

Light may be defined as energy to which the human eye is sensitive. Scientists do not yet fully understand the true nature of light in the physical sense, but the behaviour and properties of light have been extensively studied and are well known.

This book aims to describe with the aid of diagrams those aspects of optics which are relevant to the practising ophthalmologist. In this first chapter a simple account is given of the nature and properties of light.

Electromagnetic spectrum: optical radiation

Optical radiation lies between X-rays and microwaves in the electromagnetic spectrum (Fig. 1.1), and is subdivided into seven wavebands. Each of these seven wavebands group together wavelengths which elicit similar biological reactions. These seven domains are ultraviolet C (UV-C), 200–

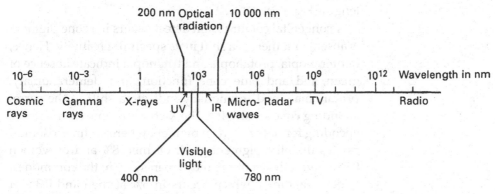

Fig. 1.1 The electromagnetic spectrum.

280 nm; ultraviolet B (UV-B), 280–315 nm; ultraviolet A (UV-A), 315–400 nm; visible radiation, 400–780 nm; infrared A (IRA), 780–1400 nm; infrared B (IRB), 1400–3000 nm; and infrared C (IRC), 3000–10000 nm. As with all electromagnetic radiation, the shorter the wavelength, the greater the energy of the individual quanta, or *photons*, of optical radiation.

The cornea and sclera of the eye absorb essentially all the incident optical radiation at very short wavelengths in the ultraviolet (UV-B and UV-C) and long wavelengths in the infrared (IR-B and IR-C). The incident UV-A is strongly absorbed by the crystalline lens while wavelengths in the range 400–1400 nm (visible light and near infrared), pass through the ocular media to fall on the retina. The visible wavelengths stimulate the retinal photoreceptors giving the sensation of light while the near infrared may give rise to thermal effects. Because the refractive surfaces of the eye focus the incident infrared radiation on the retina, it can cause retinal damage, e.g. eclipse burns.

Colour vision

The visible wavelengths of the electromagnetic spectrum are between 400 nm and 780 nm. The colour of any object is determined by the wavelengths emitted or reflected from the surface. White light is a mixture of wavelengths of the visible spectrum. Colour is perceived by three populations of cone photoreceptors in the retina which are sensitive to light of short (blue), middle (green), or long (red) wavelength (Fig. 1.2).

A congenital colour vision defect occurs if a cone pigment is absent or if there is a shift in its spectral sensitivity. Hence, deuteranopia, protanopia and tritanopia indicate absence of green, red and blue cone function, and deuteranomaly, protanomaly and tritanomaly indicate a shift in the corresponding cone sensitivity. The X-chromosome carries genes encoding for red and green pigment whereas chromosome 7 carries the blue pigment gene. Of men 8% and of women 0.5% have a defect of the red/green system; the commonest is deuteranomaly which occurs in 5% of men and 0.3% of women. Tritan defects are rare.

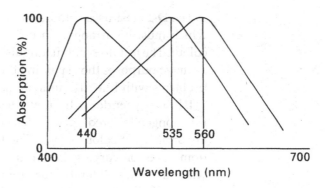

Fig. 1.2　Spectral sensitivity of cone pigments.

Congenital colour defects characteristically affect particular parts of the colour spectrum. Acquired colour defects occur throughout the spectrum but may be more pronounced in some regions. For example, acquired optic nerve disease tends to cause red–green defects. An exception occurs in glaucoma and in autosomal dominant optic neuropathy which initially cause a predominantly blue-yellow deficit; it has recently been found that visual field loss in glaucoma is detected earlier if perimetry is performed using a blue light stimulus on a yellow background. Acquired retinal disease tends to cause blue–yellow defects (except in cone dystrophy and Stargardt's disease, which cause a predominantly red–green defect).

Clinical testing of colour vision

Clinical tests of colour vision are designed to be performed in illumination equivalent to afternoon daylight in the northern hemisphere.

The **Farnsworth–Munsell (FM) hue 100** test is the most comprehensive method. It comprises 84 coloured discs, numbered in sequence on the undersurface and divided into four groups of 21. The colours of each group occupy a portion of the colour spectrum. The colours differ only in hue and have equivalent brightness and saturation. Each group must be arranged in a row with the reference colours at each end and the intervening discs in order of closest colour match. The order of placement indicates the nature of the colour defect.

The **D-15** test uses colours from all parts of the spectrum which must be arranged in order from a single reference colour. The test does not distinguish mild colour defects, but for most purposes those passing the test are unlikely to have problems with hue discrimination.

Ishihara pseudoisochromatic test plates specifically test for congenital red–green defects, the most common abnormality of colour vision. The test plates consist of random spots of varying isochromatic density. Numbers or wavy lines (for illiterates) are represented by spots of different colours. A patient who is colour blind will see only a random pattern of spots or incorrect numbers. The figures can only be distinguished from their background by their colour and not by a difference in contrast.

The **Lanthony New Colour Test** tests hue discrimination and can be used by children.

Ultraviolet light

The retinal photoreceptors are also sensitive to wavelengths between 400 nm and 350 nm in the near ultraviolet (UV-A). These wavelengths are normally absorbed by the lens of the eye. In aphakic eyes or pseudophakic eyes with intraocular implants without UV filter, such UV radiation gives rise to the sensation of blue or violet colours. Newly aphakic patients frequently remark that 'everything looks bluer than before the operation'.

Of greater concern is the recent evidence that wavebands between 350 nm in the UV and 441 nm in the visible spectrum are potentially the most dangerous for causing retinal damage under normal environmental conditions. It is therefore desirable that intraocular lenses filter out these wavelengths and protect the retina. Intraocular implant lenses are therefore being produced which incorporate a UV-A absorbing substance.

The bright illumination employed in modern ophthalmic instruments may also cause retinal damage under some circumstances. Prolonged exposure to high intensity indirect ophthalmoscope illumination, intraocular light pipe illumination and operating microscope light is potentially damaging to the retina, which may in many instances already be unhealthy. Some instruments have yellow filters built into them to reduce exposure to the most damaging wavelengths.

Fluorescence

Fluorescence is the property of a molecule to spontaneously emit light of a longer wavelength when stimulated by light of a shorter wavelength. For example, the orange dye fluorescein sodium when excited by blue light (465–490 nm) emits yellow–green light (520–530 nm) (see Fig. 1.3).

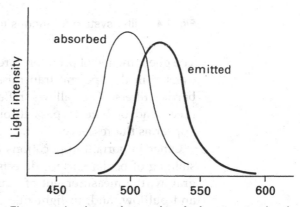

Fluorescein absorption and emission spectra (nm)

Fig. 1.3 Absorption and emission spectra of fluorescein.

Fluorescein angiography allows the state of retinal and choroidal circulation to be studied by photographing the passage of fluorescein through the vasculature after it has been administered systemically. White light from the flash unit of a fluorescein camera passes through a blue 'excitation' filter to illuminate the fundus with blue light (Fig. 1.4). The wavelengths transmitted by the excitation filter approximate to the absorption spectrum of fluorescein. Most of the light is absorbed, some is reflected unchanged, and some is changed to yellow–green light by fluorescence. The blue reflected light and yellow–green fluorescent light leaving the eye are separated by a yellow–green 'barrier' filter in the camera. This blocks blue light and exposes the camera film only to yellow–green light from the fluorescein, thereby delineating vascular structures and leakage of dye.

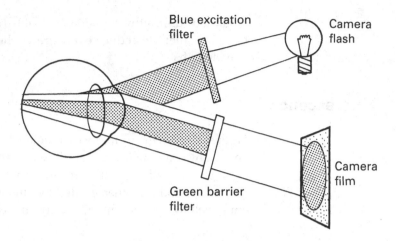

Fig. 1.4   Filter system for fundus fluorescein angiography.

The phenomenon of pseudofluorescence occurs if there is an overlap in the spectral transmission of the excitation and barrier filters. This allows reflected wavelengths at the green end of blue to pass through the barrier filter and appear as fluorescence.

Other important applications of fluorescein include the staining of ocular surface defects, anterior segment angiography, the measurement of aqueous humour production and outflow, and, in light microscopy, the localisation of tissue constituents using fluorescein bound to specific immunoglobulin.

Indocyanine green

Indocyanine green (ICG) dye is a fluorescent substance which absorbs 805 nm and emits 835 nm infrared radiation. The retinal pigment epithelium does not absorb these wavelengths, and it is therefore possible to observe fluorescence of the choroidal circulation after ICG is administered intravenously. Only 4% of 805 nm radiation absorbed by ICG is emitted at 835 nm compared with the total fluorescence of fluorescein. ICG angiography is not yet in general clinical use, but it has been shown to delineate occult choroidal neovascularisation not visible with fluorescein. ICG has also been used to photosensitise vascular lesions to diode laser photocoagulation (cf. diode laser, pp. 223–24).

Wave theory of light

The path of light through an optical medium, e.g. glass, is always straight if no obstacle or interface between optical media is encountered. Diagrammatically light is represented as a straight arrowed line or ray. (By tradition optical diagrams show rays travelling from left to right on the page.) However, some experimental observations of the behaviour of light are not fully explained by the simple concept of light as rays, and it is now understood that light really travels as waves although its path is often represented as a 'ray'.

Figure 1.5 illustrates the different ways of depicting the progress of light away from a point source. Figure 1.5a shows the light as rays; Fig. 1.5b shows the wave motion of each ray, while Fig. 1.5c illustrates the wave front set up by the combined effect of many rays, the concentric circles being drawn through the crests of the waves. The same effect is seen if a stone is dropped into still water. Viewed from above, circular waves travel outwards from the point of impact (wave fronts in Fig. 1.5c). If the process were viewed in cross-section, the waves would appear as ripples travelling away from the centre of disturbance (wave motion in Fig. 1.5b).

Wave motion consists of a disturbance, or energy, passing through a medium. The medium itself does not move, but its constituent particles vibrate at right angles to the direc-

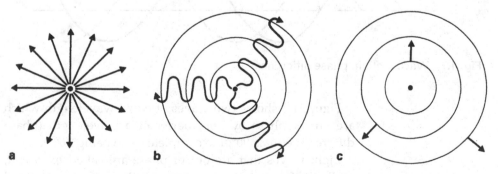

a   b   c

Fig. 1.5 Light leaving a point source. (a) Light represented as rays; (b) light represented as waves; (c) light represented as wave fronts.

tion of travel of the wave (Fig. 1.6). (Imagine a ribbon tied to a rope along which a wave is 'thrown'. The crest of the wave moves along the length of the rope, but the ribbon moves up and down at one point on the rope.)

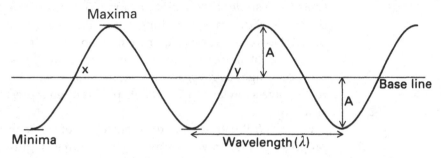

Fig. 1.6 Wave motion.

The *wavelength*, λ, is defined as the distance between two symmetrical parts of the wave motion. One complete oscillation is called a *cycle*, e.g. x y, Fig. 1.6, and occupies one wavelength. The *amplitude*, A, is the maximum displacement of an imaginary particle on the wave from the base line. Any portion of a cycle is called a *phase*. If two waves of equal wavelength (but not necessarily of equal amplitude) are travelling in the same direction but are 'out of step' with each other, the fraction of a cycle or wavelength by which one leads the other is known as the *phase difference* (Fig. 1.7).

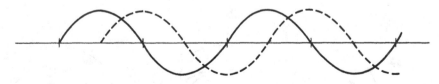

Fig. 1.7 Wave motion: phase difference.

Figure 1.7 shows two waves of equal wavelength which are out of phase by one-quarter of a wavelength (phase difference equals 90°, the complete cycle being 360°).

Light waves that are out of phase are called *incoherent*, while light composed of waves exactly in phase is termed *coherent*.

Interference

When two waves of light travel along the same path, the effect produced depends upon whether or not the waves are in phase with one another. If they are in phase, the resultant wave will be a summation of the two, and this is called *constructive interference* (Fig. 1.8a). If the two waves of equal amplitude are out of phase by half a cycle (Fig. 1.8b), they will cancel each other out: *destructive interference*. The final effect in each case is as if the waves were superimposed and added (in the algebraic sense) to each other. Phase differences of less than half a cycle thus result in a wave of intermediate amplitude and phase (Fig. 1.8c).

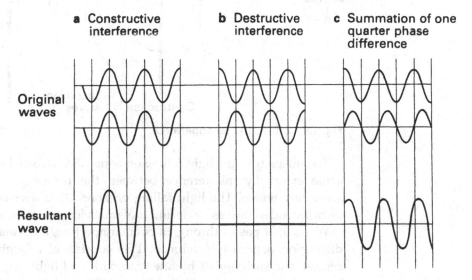

Fig. 1.8   Interference of two waves.

Destructive interference occurs within the stroma of the cornea. The collagen bundles of the stroma are so spaced that any light deviated by them is eliminated by destructive interference.

Interference phenomena are also utilised in optical instruments. One example is low reflection coatings which are applied to lens surfaces. The coating consists of a thin layer of transparent material of appropriate thickness. Light reflected from the superficial surface of the layer and light reflected from the deep surface of the layer eliminate each other by destructive interference (*cf.* Fig. 7.11).

Diffraction

When a wave front encounters a narrow opening or the edge of an obstruction (Fig. 1.9), the wave motion spreads out on the far side of the obstruction. It is as if the edge of the obstruction acts as a new centre from which secondary wave fronts are produced which are out of phase with the primary waves. This phenomenon is called *diffraction*.

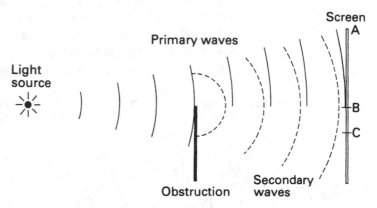

Fig. 1.9 Diffraction (exaggerated).

The intensity of the light falling on zone AB is reduced to some extent by interference between the primary and secondary waves. The light falling on zone BC is derived from secondary waves alone and is of much lower intensity.

When light passes through a circular aperture, a circular diffraction pattern is produced. This consists of a bright central disc surrounded by alternate dark and light rings. The central bright zone is known as the *Airy disc*.

Diffraction effects are most marked with small apertures, and occur in all optical systems including lenses, optical instruments and the eye. In the case of lenses and instruments, the diffraction effect at the apertures used is negligible compared with the other errors or aberrations of the system (see Chapter 8). In the case of the eye, diffraction is the main source of image imperfection when the pupil is small. However, the advantage of a large pupil in reducing diffraction is outweighed by the increased effect of the aberrations of the refractive elements of the eye (Chapter 8).

The principle of diffraction is used in the design of some multifocal intraocular lenses (pp. 138, 139).

Limit of resolution; resolving power

The terms *limit of resolution* and *resolving power* refer to the smallest angle of separation (w) between two points which allows the formation of two discernible images by an optical system (Fig. 1.10). The limit of resolution is reached when two Airy discs are separated so that the centre of one falls on the first dark ring of the other.

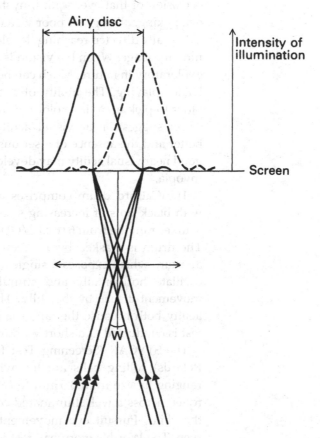

Fig. 1.10 Angle of resolution (w).

Tests of visual acuity – resolving power of the eye

It is important in clinical practice to be able to measure the resolving power of the eye. There are many tests of visual acuity. The more commonly used and important ones are discussed here. In young children, tests appropriate to the age and development of the child must be selected. As soon as the child is old enough, tests to which the response is behavioural should be replaced by those requiring matching.

Babies are best examined when alert and not hungry. Fixation with either eye should be central, steady and maintained (CSM). The best target is a face (especially that of the mother), a toy, or a television cartoon. A strong preference for one eye, indicated by an aversive response to occlusion of that eye, squint, nystagmus, roving gaze, and eye poking, all suggest poor visual acuity.

Visually directed reaching develops between two and five months of age. When the vision is poor, the movements are exploratory in nature. Much can be deduced from watching babies playing. The ability of a child aged 15 months or older to pick up a tiny coloured 'hundreds and thousands' sweet suggests near visual acuity equivalent to 6/24 or better and the absence of a serious visual defect. However, good near visual acuity may develop in the presence of high myopia.

The Catford drum comprises a white cylinder marked with black dots of increasing size corresponding to visual acuities ranging from 6/6 to 2/60 when viewed from 60 cm. The drum is masked by a screen except for a rectangular aperture which exposes a single spot. This spot is made to oscillate horizontally and stimulates corresponding eye movement if seen by the child. This test overestimates the acuity both because the target is moving and because the test is conducted at a short working distance.

The STYCAR (Screening Test for Young Children And Retards) rolling balls are ten white polystyrene spheres ranging in size from 3.5 mm to 6 cm in diameter. They are rolled across a well illuminated contrasting floor 3 m from the child. Pursuit eye movements indicate that they are seen. The Worth's ivory ball test is similar.

Other methods for assessing visual acuity in preverbal children depend upon preferential looking and the measurement of visually evoked potentials. Preferential looking can be used to assess the visual acuity of infants based upon their turning their head or eyes towards a patterned rather than a uniform target. A black and white square wave grating (alternating black and white stripes) is presented simultaneously with a plain grey target of equal size and average luminance. Children with better vision are able to see a finer grating and turn towards it.

Visual evoked potentials are the electrical responses generated in the occipital cortex by visual stimulation of the eye. The stimulus used is either a black and white square wave grating or a chequerboard pattern in which the pattern reverses at a set frequency.

An optotype is a symbol, the identification of which corresponds to a certain level of visual acuity. All tests employ black letters or pictures on an opaque or retro-illuminated white background in order to maximise contrast. The requirements of each optotype test correspond to the literary ability of the subject.

Testing of young children requires them to match the optotype letter or symbol on a card shown by the examiner who is 6 m or 3 m away by pointing to one of a group of matching letters on a key card. Children aged 18–24 months may be able to perform a picture optotype test. The Kay's pictures test uses pictures of objects such as a cat, train or house; the Cardiff cards also use pictures. The STYCAR letter tests use the letters first recognised by children (H, O, T, V and X) to test children up to the age of approximately 3 years. The Sheridan–Gardiner test uses seven letters, adding U and A.

Optotype testing of the literate involves the naming of letters. The Snellen visual acuity test is the most commonly used. The test is based on the theory that the smallest object which can be resolved by the eye subtends the same visual angle at the nodal point of the eye as a cone photoreceptor, i.e. one minute of arc (see Fig. 1.11). The test employs a chart with rows of letters of diminishing size. Each row is accorded a number indicating the distance in metres at

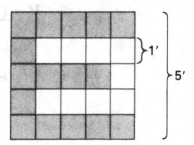

Fig. 1.11 Snellen test type letter.

which a person with normal visual acuity should correctly identify the letters. The bars and spaces of each letter subtend an angle of one minute of a degree. The test chart is normally read from 6 m (20 feet). Thus, a subject who identifies the letters on the '12' line from 6 m has 6/12 vision (20/40) – the numerator indicates the viewing distance. 'Normal' visual acuity is 6/6 (20/20) although young adults often achieve 6/4 acuity. Children are sometimes able to perform the test before 5 years of age, and may be able to match the letters to a key card before 4 years of age.

LogMAR (LOGarithm of the Minimal Angle of Resolution) visual acuity charts (e.g. the Bailey–Lovie test) are more precise than the Snellen test because they have a regular progression in the size and spacing of the letters from one line to the next and the same number of letters on every line (Fig. 1.12). Comparable results are therefore possible at any test distance.

Vernier acuity is the smallest offset of a line (Fig. 1.13)

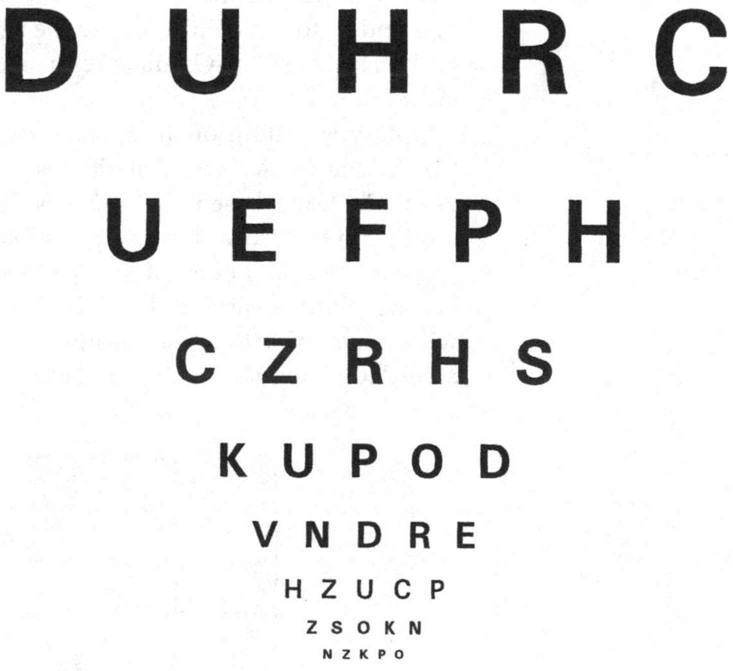

D U H R C

U E F P H

C Z R H S

K U P O D

V N D R E

H Z U C P

Z S O K N

N Z K P O

Fig. 1.12 LogMAR chart for testing visual acuity.

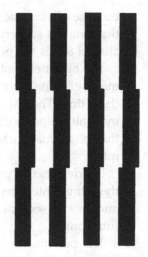

Fig. 1.13 Offset square wave grating used to measure vernier visual acuity.

which can be detected. It is measured using a square wave grating. An offset of 3–5 seconds of arc is normally discernible. This is less than the limit of Snellen visual acuity and is therefore also called hyperacuity.

Near visual acuity testing

The near visual acuity is usually tested at a distance of 25–33 cm. Near acuity charts usually comprise unrelated words or passages of text.

The British N system is based on the use of the typesetters' point system to specify the size of the metal block on which letters were traditionally cast. Each point is equal to 1/72 inch and blocks are sized in multiples of this, e.g. the blocks bearing N5 letters measure 5/72 inches in height. Times Roman is used as the standard font because the size of printed text depends on the font chosen. Jaeger text types are a less satisfactory alternative because they do not follow a logical progression in size.

Potential visual acuity testing

These tests may be used to assess the potential visual acuity of eyes in which it is not possible to see the macula e.g.

because of a cataract. Good potential visual acuity indicates that cataract surgery is likely to be of benefit. The simplest clinical test is the pinhole test. (p. 116).

The blue field entoptic phenomenon is the ability to see moving white dots when blue light diffusely illuminates the retina. They are thought to represent light transmitted by white blood cells in the perifoveal capillaries. When this phenomenon is present, macular function is grossly intact.

Interferometers project laser light from two sources on to the retina. Interference occurs where the two sources meet and this is seen as a sine wave grating if the macula is functioning.

The potential acuity meter projects a letter chart on to the retina through a small aperture (cf. pin-hole test, p. 117).

Contrast sensitivity

Tests of visual acuity do not adequately reflect the ability of the eye to see low-contrast objects such as faces. In many conditions, e.g. cataract, glaucoma and optic neuritis, the visual acuity may be almost normal whilst the contrast sensitivity is considerably reduced.

Contrast sensitivity is measured using a sine wave grating. This is a pattern in which there is a gradual transition between alternating light and dark bands, i.e. the edges of the bands appeared blurred. Narrower bands are described as having a higher spatial frequency. A contrast sensitivity curve is constructed by plotting a range of different spatial frequencies against the lowest degree of contrast at which the eye can still detect the grating. Low or very high spatial frequencies must have higher levels of contrast in order to be seen.

In clinical practice, the contrast sensitivity is measured using either a television monitor or a chart. The Pelli–Robson contrast test chart displays letters that have decreasing levels of contrast to their background. The VISITECH chart has 40 circles with different sine wave gratings and levels of contrast. The subject must indicate the orientation of the circles.

Glare testing

Scattered light which reduces visual function is called glare. Glare may be the predominant symptom of corneal oedema or scarring, cataracts or opacification of the posterior lens capsule. The effect of a glare source depends on its position and intensity and on the light scattering properties of the ocular media. Glare testing refers to the measurement of visual function (e.g. visual acuity, contrast sensitivity, colour vision) in the presence of a source of glare.

Polarisation of light

The orientation of the plane of the wave motion of rays comprising a beam of light is random unless the light is polarised. Figure 1.14a shows a beam cut across and viewed end-on: the light is travelling perpendicular to the page. In contrast, Fig. 1.14b shows the cross section of a beam of light in which the individual wave motions are lying parallel to each other. Such a beam is said to be *polarized*.

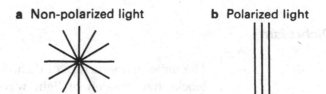

a Non-polarized light   **b Polarized light**

Fig. 1.14 Cross section of beam of light to show plane of wave motion.

Polarized light is produced from ordinary light by an encounter with a polarizing substance or agent. Polarizing substances, e.g. calcite crystals, only transmit light rays which are vibrating in one particular plane. Thus only a proportion of incident light is transmitted onward and the emerging light is polarised. A polarising medium reduces radiant intensity but does not affect spectral composition.

Light is polarised on reflection from a plane surface,

such as water, if the angle of incidence is equal to the polarising angle for the substance. The polarising angle is dependent on the refractive index of the substance comprising the reflecting surface (cf Chapters 2 and 3). At other angles of incidence the reflected light is partly polarised, i.e. a mixture of polarised and non-polarised light. Furthermore, the plane of polarisation of the reflected light from such a surface is parallel with the surface. As most reflecting surfaces encountered in daily life are horizontal, it is possible to prepare polarised sunglasses to exclude selectively the reflected horizontal polarised light (see below). Such glasses are of great use in reducing glare from the sea or wet roads.

Birefringence

Some substances have a molecular structure which transmits light waves lying parallel to its structure but which selectively slows and therefore redirects (cf. p. 33, refraction) light waves vibrating in a plane perpendicular to its structure. Crystals of quartz have this property, which is known as birefringence. Because they split incident unpolarised light into two polarised beams travelling in different directions, they have two refractive indices.

Dichroism

The molecular structure of dichroic substances completely blocks transmission of light waves not aligned with its structure by absorption. Thus, only one beam of polarised light emerges, much weakened in intensity compared with the incident non-polarised light. Tourmaline and polaroid (the latter made from fine iodine and quinine sulphate crystals embedded in plastic) are dichroic substances, polaroid being commonly used in sunglasses.

Other examples of the use of polarised light in ophthalmology are the assessment of binocular vision in which polarising glasses may be used to dissociate the eyes, e.g. in the Titmus test (p. 19); in pleoptics to produce Haidinger's brushes; and in the manufacture of optical lenses to examine them for stress.

Stereoscopic vision

Stereopsis is the ability to fuse slightly dissimilar images, which stimulate disparate retinal elements within Panum's fusional areas in the two eyes, with the perception of depth. It is graded according to the least horizontal disparity of retinal image that evokes depth perception, and is measured in seconds of arc.

The normal stereoacuity is approximately 60 seconds of arc or better (slightly different values are quoted by different workers). An individual with very good stereoscopic vision may have a stereoacuity of better than 15 seconds of arc, which is the smallest disparity offered in the Frisby stereotest (range 600–15 seconds of arc). The maximum stereoacuity is achieved when the images fall on the macular area of the retina, where the resolving power of the eye is at its best. Good stereoacuity is therefore a product of central single binocular vision. A stereoacuity of better than 250 seconds of arc is said to exclude significant amblyopia, while a stereoacuity of worse than 250 seconds of arc may be an indicator of amblyopia.

Clinical tests of stereoacuity

There are quite a variety of tests of stereoacuity available, but those most commonly used in the UK are the Titmus test, the TNO test, the Frisby test and the Lang stereotest.

The *Titmus test*, which includes the Wirt fly test, is in the form of vectographs. A vectograph consists of two superimposed views presented in such a way that the light entering each eye is plane polarised, the light from one view being at right angles to that from the other. The composite picture must be viewed through a polarising visor or spectacles.

The Wirt fly is the largest target in the test, which also includes graded sets of animals and circles, one of which is disparate and appears to stand forward. The test must be viewed at 40 cm, and covers a range of stereoacuity from approximately 3000 to 40 seconds of arc.

The *Frisby test* consists of three clear plastic plates of different thicknesses. On each plate there are four squares filled with small random shapes. One square on each plate contains a 'hidden' circle, which is printed on the back surface of the plate. The random shapes give no visual clue to the edge of the 'hidden' circle, and the test is purely three-dimensional and does not require polarising or coloured glasses to be worn. At a 40 cm viewing distance the plates show a disparity of 340, 170 and 55 seconds of arc, and by adjusting the viewing distance the test can be used to give a disparity range from 600 to 15 seconds of arc.

The *TNO test* comprises computer-generated random dot anaglyphs. An anaglyph is a stereogram in which two disparate views are printed in red and green respectively on a white ground. Red–green spectacles are worn to view the anaglyph. The eye looking through the red filter sees only the green picture, as black, and the eye looking through the green filter sees the red picture, again as black, and the two views may be fused to give a stereoscopic effect. In the TNO test the disparities range from 480 to 15 seconds of arc.

The *Lang stereotest* targets are made up of fine vertical lines which are seen alternately by each eye when focused through built-in cylindrical lens elements. The displacement of the random dot images creates disparity ranging from 1200 to 550 seconds of arc. The test card must be held parallel to the plane of the patient's face to avoid giving uniocular clues. The test is viewed at a normal reading distance.

Quantitative measurement of light (radiometry, photometry)

This topic can be confusing because of the different nomenclatures that are used. Radiometry quantifies radiant energy in all parts of the electromagnetic spectrum as an absolute value, whereas photometry quantifies part of the spectrum in terms of the visual response it produces, i.e. the spectral sensitivity of the eye. Photometric measurements are therefore more commonly employed in visual science.

Radiometry measures light in terms of how much is emitted from a source (radiant flux), its intensity (radiant intensity) and the amount falling on a surface (irradiance) or reflected from it (radiance). The equivalent photometric

measurements are luminous flux, luminous intensity, illuminance and luminance (Fig. 1.15). Radiometric and photometric units are related by the *luminous efficiency* of the
radiation, a conversion factor specific for each wavelength
determined by the sensitivity of the eye to it. The peak
photopic sensitivity of the eye is to the wavelength of
555 nm (yellow–green), at which 1 watt of monochromatic
light has a photometric equivalent of 685 lumens (see
below). This wavelength is therefore said to have maximum
luminous efficiency. The eye is progressively less sensitive
to wavelengths towards each end of the visible spectrum. In
other words, the luminous efficiency of the radiation
becomes lower and the same energy flux (radiometric unit)
is equivalent to a lower luminous flux (photometric unit).
The conversion factor falls towards zero outside the range
400–700 nm (visible light). The photometric equivalent of
polychromatic light is calculated by summating the photometric equivalents of the constituent wavelengths. The
various units are defined below.

The total flow of light emitted in all directions from a
source is termed either the *radiant flux*, if measured in watts,
or *luminous flux*, if measured in *lumens* (Fig. 1.15).

The intensity of light emitted from a source is a
measurement of the flow of light per unit solid angle of
space extending away from it. It is called either the *radiant
intensity* if measured in watts per steradian or *luminous
intensity* if measured in *candelas* (lumens per steradian). A
steradian is the unit of solid angle (resembling a cone) and
defined as the angle at the centre of a sphere which subtends
an area on the surface of the sphere measuring the square of
the radius (r). Since the surface area of a sphere is $4\pi r^2$, it
follows that a point source whose luminous intensity is one
candela emits a total of 4π lumens.

The original unit of luminous intensity was the candle,
based on the emission from a wax candle of standard
composition. Attempts to produce a more uniform and
precise source of light by which others could be measured
led to the current standard unit, the candela, whereby the
luminous intensity per square centimetre of a black body
radiator at the freezing point of platinum is defined as 60
candelas because the black body radiator is 60 times
brighter than the standard candle.

When radiant flux is incident on a surface, the surface is

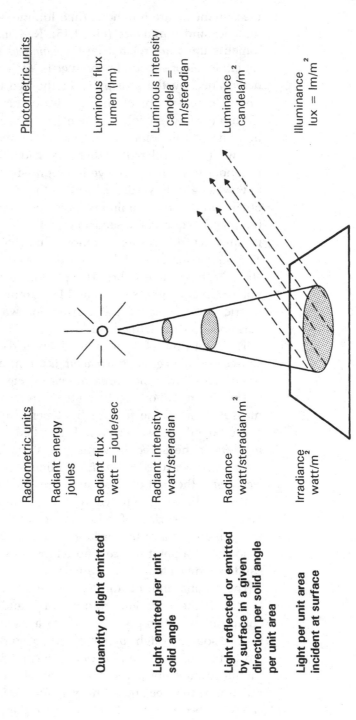

Fig. 1.15   Radiometric and photometric units of emitted and reflected light.

said to be irradiated. The flux incident per unit area at any point is called *irradiance* and is measured in watts per square metre. The photometric equivalent of irradiance is *illuminance*, which measures the luminous flux incident on an illuminated surface. The unit of illuminance is the *lux* (lumen per square metre). The illumination of a surface decreases the further it is from the light source. The surface illumination is inversely related to the square of the distance of the surface from the source (the inverse square law).

The illumination of a surface is also dependent upon the angle of the incident light to the surface. The illumination is directly related to the angle of incidence (the cosine law).

$$\text{Thus } E = \frac{I.\cos i}{d^2}$$

where E is the illumination, I is the luminous intensity, i is the angle of incidence, and d is the distance between source and surface.

A uniformly diffusing surface is one which reflects light equally in all directions. If, in addition, it reflects all the light which is incident, it is said to be a *perfect diffuser*. Each reflecting point on such a surface behaves as a point source of light because it emits light equally in all directions. The *luminance* at any point on the surface is defined as the luminous intensity per unit projected area in a given direction (Fig. 1.16a). Luminance is measured in candelas per square metre. The radiometric equivalent, *radiance*, is measured in watts per steradian per square metre. It is important to stress that the candela measures light reflected or emitted in only one direction and not the total amount leaving the surface in all directions. For most purposes, the luminance of a surface is measured not in candelas but by comparing it with a uniform diffuser which emits a total flux in all directions of 1 lumen per unit area (Fig. 1.16b). A luminous flux of one lumen per square metre corresponds to a luminance of one *apostilb*. (An alternative definition is 1 apostilb = $1/\pi$ candelas per square metre.)

Another unit, the *troland*, is a measure of retinal illumination when a surface luminance of one candela per square metre is viewed through an entrance pupil which measures one square millimetre after correction for the Stiles–Crawford effect.

a One candela per square metre

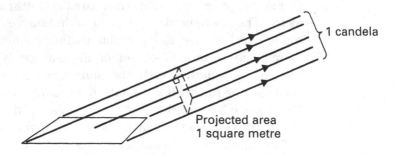

1 candela

Projected area
1 square metre

b The apostilb

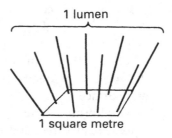

1 lumen

1 square metre

Fig. 1.16   Units of luminance.

Automated perimetry

Perimetry measures the light sensitivity of points on the retina by the ability of the patient to detect light stimuli of varying intensity presented at corresponding points in the visual field. Currently, most perimeters have a standard background luminance of 31.5 apostilbs (asb). The eye to be tested should be positioned at the centre of the hemisphere, and the near spectacle correction should be worn whilst the patient maintains steady fixation. Spots of light are projected on to the inner surface of the hemisphere.

Light stimuli may vary in intensity between 0.8 and 10 000 asb. This range can be expressed as a logarithmic scale and the log units are termed decibels (dB; 1 log unit equals 10 dB). The range 0.8–10 000 asb used in perimetry corresponds to 51 dB.

2   Reflection of Light

When light meets an interface between two media, its behaviour depends on the nature of the two media involved. Light may be absorbed by the new medium, or transmitted onward through it (see Chapter 3), or it may bounce back into the first medium. This 'bouncing' of light at an interface is called *reflection*. It occurs, to some degree, at all interfaces even when most of the light is transmitted or absorbed. It is by the small amount of reflected light that we see a glass door and thus avoid walking into it.

Laws of reflection

The following laws govern reflection of light at any interface and are illustrated in Fig. 2.1.

(1)   The incident ray, the reflected ray and the normal to the reflecting surface all lie in the same plane. (The 'normal' is a line perpendicular to the surface at the point of reflection.)

(2)   Angle of incidence, i, equals the angle of reflection, r.

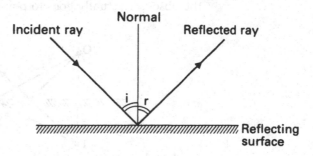

Fig. 2.1.   Reflection at a plane surface.

Reflection at an irregular surface

When parallel light encounters an irregular surface, it is scattered in many directions (Fig. 2.2). This is called diffuse reflection.

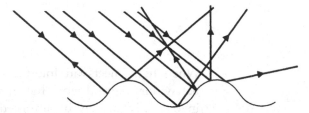

Fig. 2.2 Reflection at an irregular surface: diffuse reflection.

It is by diffuse reflection that most objects (except self-luminous ones) are seen, e.g. furniture, etc. A perfect reflecting surface (free from irregularities causing diffuse reflection) would itself be invisible. Only the image formed by light reflected in it would be seen.

Reflection at a plane surface: plane mirrors

In Fig. 2.3, light from object O is reflected at the surface according to the laws of reflection. If the reflected rays are produced behind the surface, they all intersect at point I, the image of object O.

The brain always assumes that an object is situated in the direction from which light enters the eye. Light from object O appears to come from point I, the image of O. However, if the observer actually goes to point I, there is no real image

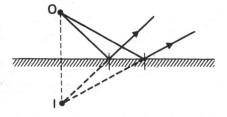

Fig. 2.3 Reflection at a plane surface: point object.

present: it could not be captured on a screen. Such images are called *virtual*. Images which can be captured on a screen are called *real* images.

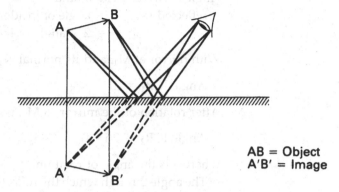

AB = Object
A'B' = Image

Fig. 2.4 Reflection at a plane surface: extended object.

The image of an object formed by reflection at a plane surface has the following characteristics. It is upright (erect), virtual, and laterally inverted. It lies along a line perpendicular to the reflecting surface and is as far behind the surface as the object is in front of it.

Rotation of a plane mirror

If a plane mirror is rotated while light is incident upon its centre of rotation, the reflected ray is deviated through an angle equal to twice the angle of rotation of the mirror.

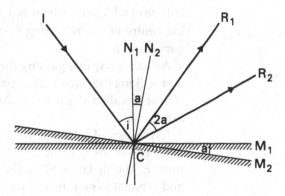

Fig. 2.5 Rotation of a plane mirror.

By the laws of reflection:

Angle of incidence = angle of reflection
Therefore
Angle between incident and
    reflected ray   = angle of incidence + angle of reflection
                 = 2 × angle of incidence

With mirror at M_1, and its normal N_1,

    Angle ICR_1 = 2i

After rotation of the mirror to M_2, with normal N_2,

    Angle ICR_2 = 2(i + a)

where a is the angle of rotation.
    The angle through which the reflected ray is deviated when the mirror rotates from M_1 to M_2 is angle R_1CR_2.
    But
$$R_1CR_2 = ICR_2 - ICR_1$$
$$= 2(i + a) - 2i$$
$$= 2a$$

Reflection at spherical reflecting surfaces

A reflecting surface having the form of a portion of a sphere is called a spherical mirror. If the reflecting surface lies on the inside of the curve, it is a *concave* mirror. If the reflecting surface lies on the outside of the curve, the mirror is a *convex* mirror.

In Fig. 2.6, the *centre of curvature*, C, is the centre of the sphere of which the mirror is a part, the *pole of the mirror*, P, is the centre of the reflecting surface, and CP = the radius of curvature, r.

An *axis* is any line passing through the centre of curvature and striking the mirror. That passing through the pole of the mirror is called the *principal axis*; any other is a *subsidiary axis*.

Rays parallel to the principal axis are reflected towards (concave) or away from (convex) the *principal focus*, F, of the mirror. The distance FP is the *focal length*, f, of the mirror and is equal to half the radius of curvature. Thus, the image of an object situated on the principal axis an infinite

a Concave mirror

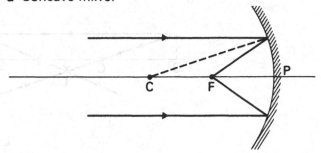

b Convex mirror

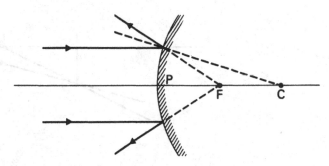

Fig. 2.6 Spherical mirror: reflection of parallel light.

distance away is formed at the principal focus (Fig. 2.6). The image formed by the concave mirror is real while that formed by the convex mirror is virtual. The following diagrams show the nature and situation of images formed of objects situated at a finite distance from the mirror on the principal axis. In each case the image is constructed using two rays:

(1) A ray parallel to the principal axis and reflected to or away from the principal focus.

(2) A ray from the top of the object, passing through the centre of curvature and reflected back along its own path.

For any position of the object, the position of the image formed by a spherical mirror can be calculated using the formula:

$$\frac{1}{v} - \frac{1}{u} = \frac{1}{f} = \frac{2}{r}$$

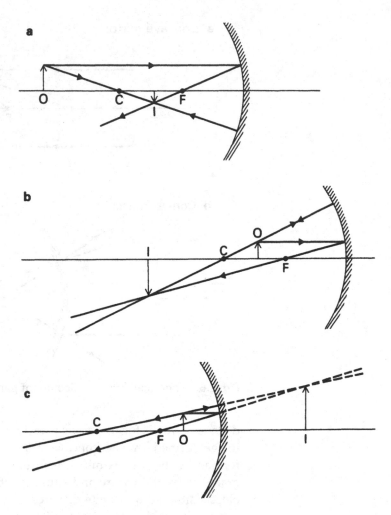

Fig. 2.7   Image formation by the concave mirror. (a) Object outside the centre of curvature, C. Image real, inverted, diminished (reduced in size), lying between C and principal focus F. (b) Object between centre of curvature C, and principal focus F. Image real, inverted, enlarged, lying outside the centre of curvature C. (c) Object inside principal focus F. Image erect, virtual and enlarged.

where u is the distance of the object from the mirror, v is the distance of the image from the mirror, f is the focal length of the mirror, and r is the radius of curvature of the mirror.

Also, the magnification produced by a curved mirror can be calculated. Magnification is defined as the ratio of image size to object size where M = magnification, i = image size,

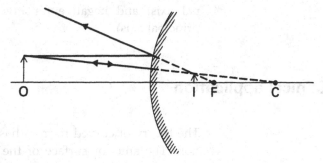

Fig. 2.8 Image formation by the convex mirror. The object may be located at any distance from the mirror. The image is virtual, erect and diminished.

and o = object size. The magnification can be calculated using the formula:

$$\frac{i}{o} = -\frac{v}{u}$$

where v is the distance of the image from the mirror, and u is the distance of the object from the mirror.

When using these formulae, the sign convention must be adhered to (Fig. 2.9).

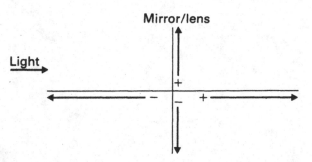

Fig. 2.9 Sign convention.

All distances are measured from the pole of the mirror (or vertex of the lens) to the point in question.

Distances measured in the same direction as the incident light are positive, those against the direction of the incident light are negative. (The incident light is usually shown coming from the left in optical diagrams.)

Image size is positive for erect images (above the principal axis) and negative for inverted images (below the principal axis).

Clinical application

The theory of curved mirrors has a major clinical application. The anterior surface of the cornea acts as a convex mirror and is used as such by the standard instruments employed to measure corneal curvature (see keratometer, Chapter 14).

Images formed by the reflecting surfaces of the eye are called catoptric images and are described in Chapter 9.

3   Refraction of Light

Refraction is defined as the change in direction of light when it passes from one transparent medium into another of different optical density. The incident ray, the refracted ray and the normal all lie in the same plane.

The velocity of light varies according to the density of the medium through which it travels. The more dense the medium the slower the light passes through it. When a beam of light strikes the interface separating a less dense medium from a denser one obliquely (Fig. 3.1), the edge of the beam which arrives first, A, is retarded on entering the denser medium.

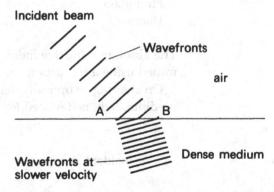

Fig. 3.1 Refraction of beam of light entering an optically dense medium from air.

The opposite side of the beam, B, is meanwhile continuing at its original velocity. The beam is thus deviated as indicated in Fig. 3.1, being bent towards the normal (the 'normal' being a line perpendicular to the interface at the point of refraction) as it enters the denser medium.

A comparison of the velocity of light in a vacuum and in

another medium gives a measure of the *optical density* of that medium. This measurement is called the *absolute refractive index*, n, of the medium.

Absolute refractive index $= {}_{vacuum}n_{medium}$

$$= \frac{\text{Velocity of light in vacuum}}{\text{Velocity of light in medium}}$$

As the optical density of air as a medium is negligible under normal conditions,

Refractive index $= {}_{air}n_{medium}$

$$= \frac{\text{Velocity of light in air}}{\text{Velocity of light in medium}}$$

Examples of refractive index are:

Air	= 1
Water (incl. Aqueous)	= 1.33
Cornea	= 1.37
Crystalline lens	= 1.386–1.406
Crown glass	= 1.52
Flint glass	= 1.6
Diamond	= 2.5

The absolute refractive index of any material can be determined using a refractometer.

On entering an optically dense medium from a less dense medium, light is deviated *towards* the normal.

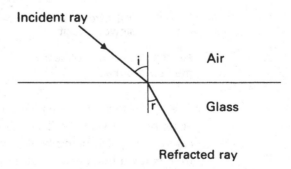

Fig. 3.2 Refraction of light entering an optically dense medium from air.

The incident ray makes an angle, i, *the angle of incidence*, with the normal. The angle between the refracted ray and the normal is called the *angle of refraction*, r.

These angles are governed by the refractive indices of the media involved according to Snell's law.

Snell's law states that the incident ray, refracted ray and the normal all lie in the same plane and that the angles of incidence, i, and refraction, r, are related to the refractive index, n, of the media concerned by the equation

$$_{medium_1}n_{medium_2} = \frac{\sin i}{\sin r}$$

where the first medium is a vacuum, n is the absolute refractive index, and in air n is the refractive index.

If, however, the interface is between two denser media of differing optical densities, e.g. water and glass, then the value of n for that interface may be calculated as follows

$$_{water}n_{glass} = \frac{n_{glass}}{n_{water}}$$

More generally, on passing from medium$_1$ into medium$_2$, the index of refraction is given by

$$_1n_2 = \frac{n_2}{n_1}$$

Light passing obliquely through a plate of glass (Fig. 3.3) is deviated laterally and the emerging ray is parallel to the incident ray. Thus the direction of the light is unchanged but it is laterally displaced.

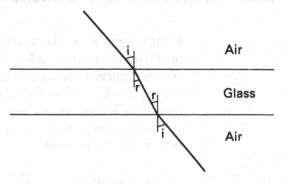

Fig. 3.3 Refraction of light through parallel-sided slab of glass.

It should be remembered that some reflection also occurs at every interface (Chapter 2) even though in this case most of the incident light passes onwards by refraction. For example, a lens or window with a refractive index of 1.5 in air reflects 4% of light from the anterior surface and transmits the remaining 96% to the posterior surface; a further 4% of this is reflected so that the lens transmits only 92.16% of normally incident light (cf. pp. 9, 87, lens coatings).

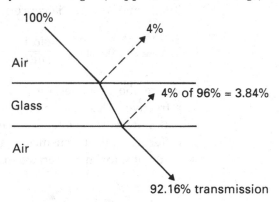

Fig. 3.4 Reflection and transmission of light by transparent media.

Figure 3.5 illustrates the use of a sheet of glass as an image-splitter, e.g. the teaching mirror of the indirect ophthalmoscope. Most of the light is refracted across the glass to the examiner's eye. However, a small proportion is reflected at the anterior surface of the glass and enables an observer to see the same view as the examiner.

Refraction of light at a curved interface

Light passing across a curved interface between two media of different refractive indices obeys Snell's law. A convex spherical curved surface causes parallel light to converge to a focus if n_2 is greater than n_1, or to diverge as from a point focus if n_2 is less than n_1 (Fig. 3.6).

The refracting power or vergence power of such a surface is given by the formula

$$\text{Surface power} = \frac{n_2 - n_1}{r}$$

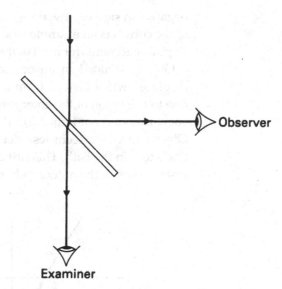

Fig. 3.5 Parallel-sided glass sheet used as an image-splitter.

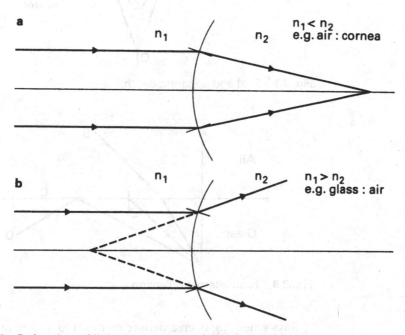

Fig. 3.6 Refraction of light at a convex refracting interface, e.g. cornea.

where r is the radius of curvature of the surface in metres according to the sign convention (see p. 31) and the surface power is measured in dioptres (see p. 59).

Surface power is positive for converging surfaces and

negative in sign for diverging surfaces. The anterior surface of the cornea is an example of such a refracting surface, and its power accounts for most of the refracting power of the eye.

Objects situated in an optically dense medium appear displaced when viewed from a less dense medium. This is due to refraction of the emerging rays which now appear to come from a point I, the virtual image of object O (Fig. 3.7). Objects in water seem less deep than they really are, e.g. one's toes in the bath. This principle applies also to surgical instruments in the anterior chamber of the eye.

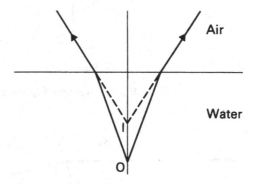

Fig. 3.7 Real and apparent depth.

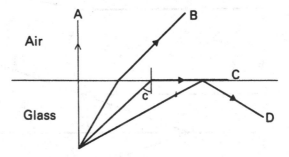

Fig. 3.8 Total internal reflection.

Rays emerging from a denser medium to a rarer medium suffer a variety of fates, depending on the angle at which they strike the interface. Ray A strikes at 90° to the interface and is undeviated. Ray B emerges after refraction. As the rays meet the interface more obliquely, a stage is reached where the refracted ray, Ray C, runs parallel with the interface. The angle c is called the *critical angle*. Rays striking more obliquely still fail to emerge from the denser medium and are reflected back into it as from a mirror. This is called *total internal reflection*.

The critical angle is determined by the refractive indices of the media involved and can be calculated using Snell's law. The critical angle for the tear film/air interface is 48.5°, and for a crown glass/air interface the critical angle is 41°.

Total internal reflection is used in optical instruments. Prisms make excellent reflectors by total internal reflection (Chapter 4, pp. 41, 42). Fibre optic cables, which are used to deliver light from a remote source to the point where it is required, also depend on total internal reflection. Examples include the surgical intraocular light source and the transmission of laser light from the laser tube to the delivery system of the laser slit lamp.

Fibre optic cables consist of many fine transparent fibres bound together in a flexible external protective sheath. Light enters the end of each fibre and is reflected onward by total internal reflection until it emerges from the far end without significant loss of radiant energy (Fig. 3.9). Bending the optical fibre does not impair its efficiency.

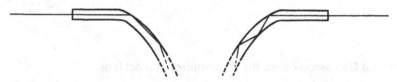

Fig. 3.9 Total internal reflection – single fibre of fibre optic cable.

Total internal reflection also occurs at surfaces within the eye, notably the cornea:air interface, and prevents visualisation of parts of the eye, e.g. the angle of the anterior chamber and peripheral retina. The problem is overcome by applying a contact lens made of material with a higher refractive index than the eye and filling the space between

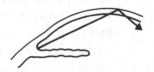

Fig. 3.10 Total internal reflection at the cornea of light from the angle of the anterior chamber.

eye and lens with saline, thus destroying the cornea/air refracting surface and allowing visualisation of the anterior chamber angle (gonioscopy) and peripheral retina (three-mirror).

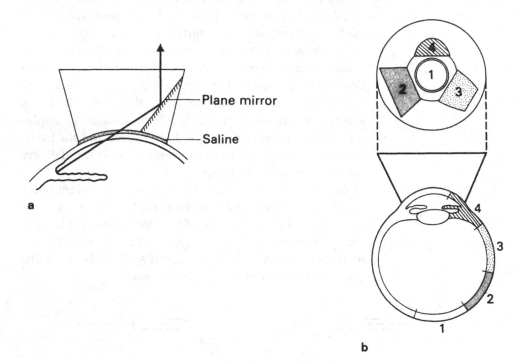

Fig. 3.11 (a) Gonioscopy lens. (b) Three-mirror contact lens.

Dispersion of light

So far, this discussion of refraction has overlooked the fact that white light is composed of various wavelengths. In fact, the refractive index of any medium differs slightly for light of different wavelengths.

Light of shorter wavelength is deviated more than light of longer wavelength, e.g. blue light is deviated more than red. The refractive index of a material is normally taken to mean that for the yellow sodium flame.

The angle formed between the red and blue light around the yellow (Fig. 3.12) indicates the *dispersive power* of the medium (cf. chromatic aberration, p. 89). This is not related to the refractive index of the material.

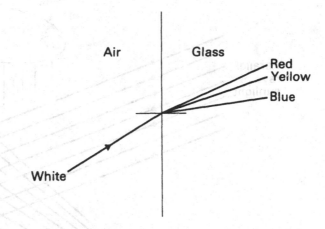

Fig. 3.12 Diagram to show dispersion of light. (The angles involved are exaggerated.)

The rainbow: total internal reflection and dispersion

When sunlight enters a raindrop it is dispersed into its constituent spectral colours (Fig. 3.13). Under certain circumstances, the angle of incidence is such that total internal reflection then occurs within the drop. The dispersed light finally emerges, each wavelength or colour making a different angle with the horizon. To see the rainbow, the observer must look away from the sun.

The observer receives only a narrow pencil of rays from each drop, i.e. only one colour. The whole rainbow is the result of rays received from a bank of drops at increasing angle to the observer's eye (see Fig. 3.14). Violet, the colour

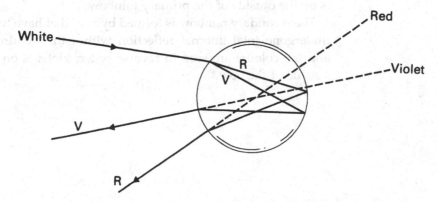

Fig. 3.13 Formation of the primary rainbow. Path of light within one raindrop.

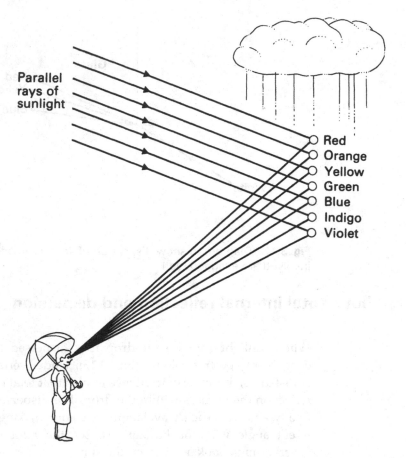

Fig. 3.14 Formation of primary rainbow (composite diagram).

making the smallest angle to the horizon, is received from the lower drops while red, making the greatest angle with the horizon, is received from the highest drops. Thus the red is on the outside of the primary rainbow.

The secondary rainbow is formed by rays that have twice undergone total internal reflection within the raindrops, and the colours are seen in reverse order: violet is on the outside of the bow.

4   Prisms

A prism is defined as a portion of a refracting medium bordered by two plane surfaces which are inclined at a finite angle. The angle α between the two surfaces is called the *refracting angle* or *apical angle* of the prism (Fig. 4.1). A line bisecting the angle is called the axis of the prism. The opposite surface is called the *base* of the prism. When prescribing prisms, the orientation is indicated by the position of the base, e.g. 'base-in', 'base-up'.

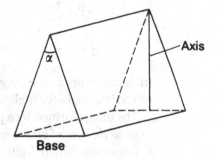

Fig. 4.1 Prism. The refracting angle (α).

Light passing through a prism (Fig. 4.2) obeys Snell's law at each surface. The ray is deviated towards the base of the prism. The net change in direction of the ray, angle D, is called the *angle of deviation*.

For a prism in air, the angle of deviation is determined by three factors:

(1) The refractive index of the material of which the prism is made.
(2) The refracting angle, α, of the prism.
(3) The angle of incidence of the ray considered.

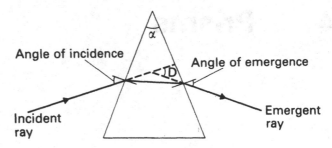

Fig. 4.2 Passage of light through a prism.

For any particular prism, the angle of deviation D is least when the angle of incidence equals the angle of emergence. Refraction is then said to be symmetrical and the angle is called the *angle of minimum deviation*. Under these conditions the angle of deviation is given by the formula

$$D = (n-1)\alpha$$

Thus, for a glass prism of refractive index 1.5,

$$D = (1.5-1)\alpha$$

$$= \frac{\alpha}{2}$$

In other words, the angle of deviation equals half the refracting angle for a glass prism.

The image formed by a prism is erect, virtual and *displaced towards the apex of the prism* (Fig. 4.3). Deviation is reduced to a minimum when light passes through the prism symmetrically.

There are two primary positions in which the power of a prism may be specified, the position of minimum deviation

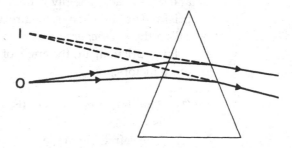

Fig. 4.3 Image formation by a prism.

and the Prentice position. In the Prentice position one surface of the prism is normal to the ray of light so that all the
deviation takes place at the other surface of the prism (Fig.
4.4).

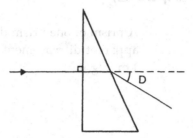

Fig. 4.4 The Prentice position of a prism.

The deviation of light in the Prentice position is greater
than that in the position of minimum deviation, because in
the Prentice position the angle of incidence does not equal
the angle of emergence. Therefore the Prentice position
power of any prism is greater than its power in the position
of minimum deviation.

It is the Prentice position power which is normally
specified for glass ophthalmic prisms, e.g. trial lens prisms,
while it is the power in the position of minimum deviation
which is specified for plastic ophthalmic prisms, e.g. prism
bars. If a high-power prism is not used in the correct position, a considerable error will result. In practice, plastic
prisms may be held in the frontal plane as this is near
enough to the position of minimum deviation to avoid
significant inaccuracy. For example, a 40 dioptre plastic
prism held in the frontal plane will have an effective power
of 41 dioptres, but if it is held in the Prentice position its
effective power becomes 72 dioptres.

Furthermore, it is not satisfactory to stack prisms one on
top of another, because the light entering the second and
subsequent prisms will not be at the correct angle of incidence. The effective power of such a stack will be significantly different from the sum of the powers of the
component prisms. However, it is permissible to place a
horizontal and a vertical prism one in front of the other,
because their planes of refraction are perpendicular and
therefore independent of one another.

Notation of prisms

The power of any prism can be expressed in various units.

The prism dioptre (Δ)

A prism of one prism dioptre power (1^Δ) produces a linear apparent displacement of 1 cm, of an object O, situated at 1 m (Fig. 4.5).

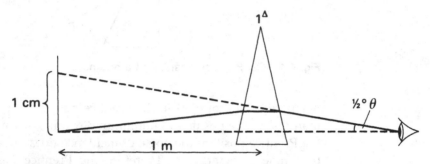

Fig. 4.5   The prism dioptre and angle of apparent deviation (θ).

Angle of apparent deviation

The apparent displacement of the object O can also be measured in terms of the angle θ, the angle of apparent deviation (Fig. 4.5). Under conditions of ophthalmic usage a prism of 1 prism dioptre power produces an angle of apparent deviation of $\frac{1}{2}^\circ$. Thus 1 prism dioptre $= \frac{1}{2}^\circ$.

The centrad (∇)

This unit differs from the prism dioptre only in that the image displacement is measured along an arc 1 m from the prism (Fig. 4.6). The centrad produces a very slightly greater angle of deviation than the prism dioptre, but the difference, in practice, is negligible.

Refracting angle

A prism may also be described by its refracting angle (Fig. 4.1). However, unless the refractive index of the prism

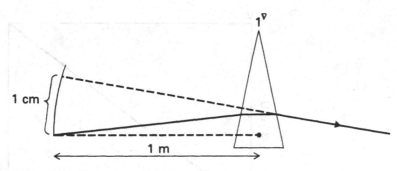

Fig. 4.6 The centrad (∇).

material is also known, the prism power cannot be deduced.

Summary of prism units

Thus a glass prism of refracting angle 10° (a ten-degree prism) deviates light through 5° and has a power of 10 prism dioptres (10^Δ), assuming its refractive index is 1.5.

Vector addition of prisms

Sometimes a patient requires a prismatic correction in both the horizontal and the vertical directions. This can conveniently be achieved by using one stronger prism mounted at an oblique angle. The required power and angle is calculated by vector addition, either graphically or mathematically (Fig. 4.7).

Graphically, the required horizontal and vertical powers are drawn to scale and the rectangle completed (Fig. 4.7). The diagonal gives the power and the angle ROH the angle required for a single equivalent prism. The orientation must be specified in terms of the angle, base up/down, and base in/out.

Mathematically, the diagonal power is calculated using Pythagoras' theorem (the square of the diagonal equals the sum of the squares of the vertical and horizontal sides) and tan ROH = RH/OH. Thus, Fig. 4.7 shows that a 5 dioptre prism base-up and in, lying in the 37° meridian, is equiva-

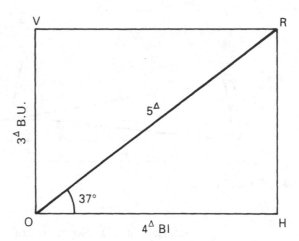

Fig. 4.7 Vector addition of prisms.

lent to a 4 dioptre base-in prism plus a 3 dioptre base-up prism.

Risley prism

The Risley prism is another application of this principle. It consists of two prisms of equal power which are mounted one in front of the other in such a way that they can be rotated with respect to each other and the resulting power is indicated on a scale on the rim of the instrument. A Risley prism may be used in conjunction with a Maddox rod (pp. 67–69) to measure phorias, and is included in the refractor heads used by many optometrists (instead of a trial lens box).

Interpretation of orthoptic reports

Armed with the knowledge that 1 prism dioptre $= \frac{1}{2}°$, orthoptic reports become intelligible to the clinician.

The orthoptist measures the angle of squint by two methods. Using the synoptophore, she measures the angle between the visual axes of the eyes in degrees, + *signifying esotropia and* – *signifying exotropia*. Her report reads

Synopt. without gls +20°

She also measures the angle of squint by the prism cover test (PCT). The alternating cover test is performed, placing prisms of increasing strength before one eye, until movement of the eyes is eliminated (Fig. 4.8). The result is expressed in prism dioptres, *eso signifying esotropia and exo signifying exotropia.* Her report reads

$$PCT = distance \; eso \; +40^{\Delta}$$

These two statements express the same angle of squint.

Use of prisms

Diagnostic prisms

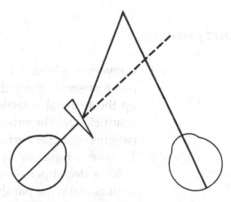

Fig. 4.8 Use of a prism in squint.

(1) Assessment of squint and heterophoria.
   (a) Measurement of angle objectively by prism cover test.
   (b) Measurement of angle subjectively by Maddox rod.
   (c) To assess likelihood of diplopia after proposed squint surgery in adults.
   (d) Measurement of fusional reserve. Increasingly powerful prisms are placed before one eye until fusion breaks down. This is very useful in assessing the presence of binocular single vision in children under 2 years of age.
   (e) The four-dioptre prism test. This is a delicate test for small degrees of esotropia (microtropia). A

four-dioptre prism placed base-out before the deviating eye causes no movement as the image remains within the suppression scotoma. When placed before the normal (fixing) eye, movement occurs.

(2) Assessment of simulated blindness. If a prism is placed in front of a seeing eye, the eye will move to regain fixation.

Forms of prism used in diagnosis

Forms of prism used in assessment include single unmounted prisms, the prisms from the trial lens set and prism bars. These are bars composed of adjacent prisms of increasing power.

Therapeutic prisms

(1) Convergence insufficiency. The commonest therapeutic use of prisms in the orthoptic department is in building up the fusional reserve of patients with convergence insufficiency. The prisms are used base-out during the patients' exercise periods. *They are not worn constantly.*

(2) To relieve diplopia in certain cases of squint. These include decompensated heterophorias, small vertical squints and some paralytic squints with diplopia in the primary position. Prisms are reserved for those patients for whom surgery is not indicated.

Forms of therapeutic prism

(1) Temporary wear. Prisms used in treatment include clip-on spectacle prisms for trial wear. An improvement on these are *Fresnel prisms*, which are available in all powers employed clinically. A Fresnel prism consists of a plastic sheet of parallel tiny prisms of identical refracting angle (Fig. 4.9). The overall prismatic effect is the same as that of a single large prism. The sheets are lighter than a glass prism and can be stuck on to the patient's glasses.

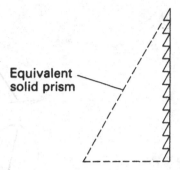

Fig. 4.9 Fresnel prism.

(2)   Permanent wear. Permanent incorporation of a prism
      into a patient's spectacles can be achieved by decen-
      tring the spherical lens already present, see p. 64.
      Alternatively, prisms can be mounted in spectacles.

Notes on prescription of prisms

Generally, when prescribing prisms, the correction is split
between the two eyes (Fig. 4.10).

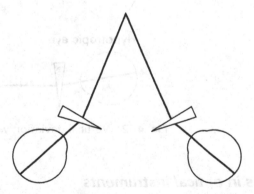

Fig. 4.10 Convergence with prismatic correction.

To correct convergence the prisms must be base-out, e.g. 8^Δ
base-out R and L (Fig. 4.10). To correct divergence the
prisms must be base-in, e.g. 6^Δ base-in R and L (Fig. 4.11). To
correct vertical deviation the orientation of the prisms is
opposite for the two eyes, e.g.

   2^Δ base-down RE
   2^Δ base-up LE for R hypertropia

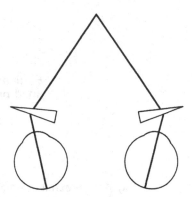

Fig. 4.11 Divergence with prismatic correction.

The apex of the prism must always be placed towards the direction of deviation of the eye (Fig. 4.12).

Hypertropic eye

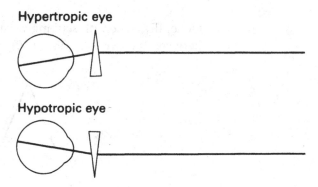

Hypotropic eye

Fig. 4.12 Vertical deviation with prismatic correction.

Prisms in optical instruments

Prisms are commonly used in ophthalmic instruments as reflectors of light. The prism is designed and orientated so that total internal reflection occurs within it.

It can be seen that prisms give greater flexibility in dealing with an image than do mirrors. There are many possible systems available (Fig. 4.13).

Instruments in which prisms are used include the slit lamp microscope, the applanation tonometer and the keratometer (see Chapter 14).

Right angle prism

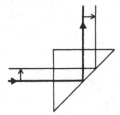

Deviation 90°

Porro prism

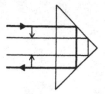

Deviation 180°
Image inverted but not
transposed left to right

Dove prism

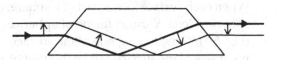

No deviation
Image inverted but not
laterally transposed

Fig. 4.13 Some prisms used in optical instruments.

5   Spherical Lenses

A lens is defined as a portion of a refracting medium bordered by two curved surfaces which have a common axis. When each surface forms part of a sphere, the lens is called a spherical lens. Various forms of spherical lens are possible (Fig. 5.1), some having one plane surface. This is acceptable because a plane surface can be thought of as part of a sphere of infinite radius.

A convex lens causes convergence of incident light, whereas a concave lens causes divergence of incident light (Fig. 5.2).

The total vergence power (Fig. 5.3) of a spherical lens depends on the vergence power of each surface (see Chapter 3, p. 36) and the thickness of the lens. Most of the lenses used in ophthalmology are thin lenses, and for a thin lens the thickness factor may be ignored. Thus the total power of a thin lens is the sum of the two surface powers. Refraction can be thought of as occurring at the principal plane of the lens, and in the following lens diagrams only the principal plane is shown. Refraction by thick lenses is more complicated, and the theory of the thick lens is dealt with in Chapter 9 as it is more relevant to the study of the refracting mechanism of the eye.

In Fig. 5.4 a and b the *principal plane* of the lens is shown, AB. (Note that in ray diagrams the convex or concave nature of a thin lens is shown by the appropriate symbol at each end of the line that indicates the principal plane.) The point at which the principal plane and principal axis intersect is called the *principal point* or *nodal point*, N, of the lens. Rays of light passing through the nodal point are undeviated.

Light parallel to the principal axis is converged to or diverged from the point F, the *principal focus* (Fig. 5.5). As the medium on both sides of the lens is the same (air), parallel

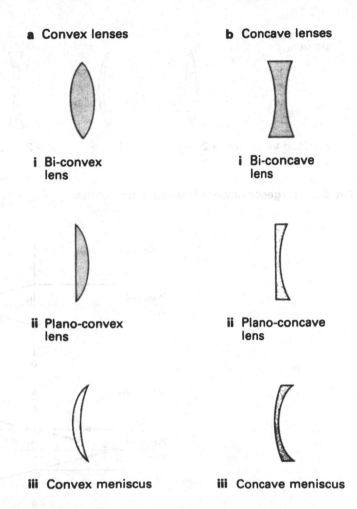

a Convex lenses

i Bi-convex lens

ii Plano-convex lens

iii Convex meniscus

b Concave lenses

i Bi-concave lens

ii Plano-concave lens

iii Concave meniscus

Fig. 5.1 Basic forms of spherical lenses.

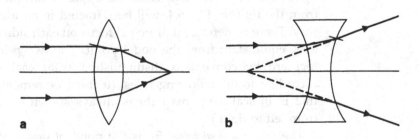

a   **b**

Fig. 5.2 Light passing through a lens obeys Snell's law at each surface. (a) Convex lens; (b) concave lens.

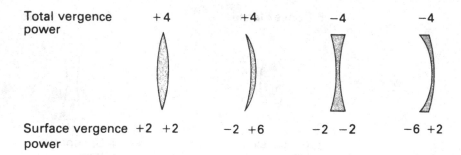

Total vergence power   +4   +4   −4   −4

Surface vergence power   +2 +2   −2 +6   −2 −2   −6 +2

Fig. 5.3   Vergence power of thin spherical lenses.

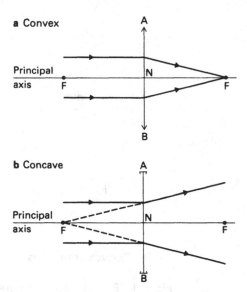

Fig. 5.4   Cardinal points of thin spherical lenses. (a) Convex; (b) concave.

light incident on the lens from the opposite direction, i.e. from the right in Fig. 5.4, will be refracted in an identical way. There is therefore a principal focus on each side of the lens, equidistant from the nodal point. The two principal foci are by convention distinguished from each other according to the following rules. (It must be remembered that in optical diagrams light is always shown travelling from left to right.)

The *first principal focus*, F_1, is the point of origin of rays which, after refraction by the lens, are parallel to the principal axis. The distance F_1N is the first focal length f_1.

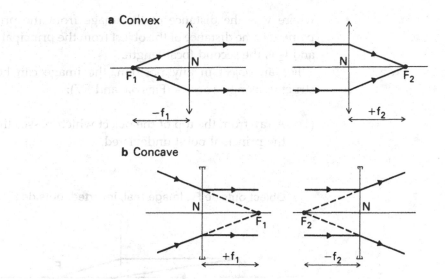

Fig. 5.5 The principal foci of thin spherical lenses.

Incident light parallel to the principal axis is converged to or diverged from the *second principal focus*, F_2. The distance F_2N is the second focal length, f_2. By the sign convention (see p. 31) f_2 has a positive sign for the convex lens, and a negative sign for the concave lens.

Lenses are designated by their second focal length. Thus, convex or converging lenses are sometimes called 'plus lenses', and are marked with a +, while concave or diverging lenses are known as 'minus lenses' and are marked with a –.

If the medium on either side of the lens is the same, e.g. air, then $f_1 = f_2$. However, if the second medium differs from the first, e.g. as in the case of a contact lens, then f_1 will not equal f_2 (cf. refraction at curved interfaces, Chapter 3).

Thin lens formula

As with spherical mirrors, the position and nature of the image formed by a spherical lens depends on the position of the object and a similar formula applies:

$$\frac{1}{v} - \frac{1}{u} = \frac{1}{f_2}$$

where v is the distance of the image from the principal point; u is the distance of the object from the principal point; and f_2 is the second focal length.

For an object in any position, the image can be constructed using two rays (Figs 5.6 and 5.7):

(1) A ray from the top of the object which passes through the principal point undeviated.

a Object outside F_1. Image real, inverted, outside F_2

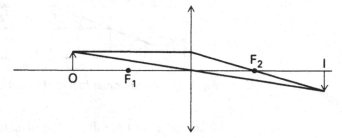

b Object at F_1. Image virtual, erect, at infinity

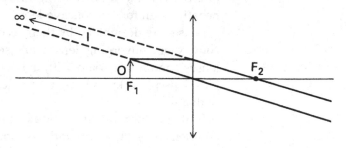

c Object inside F_1. Image virtual, erect, magnified, further from lens than object

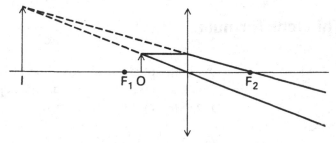

Fig. 5.6 Image formation by a thin convex lens.

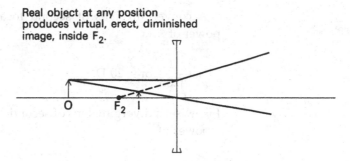

Real object at any position produces virtual, erect, diminished image, inside F_2.

Fig. 5.7 Image formation by a thin concave lens.

(2) A ray parallel to the principal axis, which after refraction passes through (convex) or away from (concave) the second principal focus.

Dioptric power of lenses. Vergence

Lenses of shorter focal length are more powerful than lenses of longer focal length. Therefore the unit of lens power, the *dioptre*, is based on the reciprocal of the second focal length. The reciprocal of the second focal length expressed in metres, gives the *vergence power* of the lens in dioptres (D) thus (Fig. 5.8):

$$F = \frac{1}{f_2}$$

where F is the vergence power of the lens in dioptres and f_2 is the second focal length *in metres*.

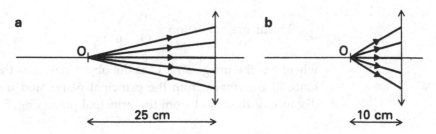

Fig. 5.8 Vergence of rays.

(a) Vergence at the lens

$$= \frac{1}{0.25}$$

$$= 4 \text{ Dioptres}$$

(b) Vergence at the lens

$$= \frac{1}{0.10}$$

$$= 10 \text{ Dioptres}$$

A converging lens of second focal length +5 cm has a power of

$$+\frac{1}{0.05} \text{ or } + 20 \text{ D.}$$

Likewise, a diverging lens of second focal length –25 cm has a power of

$$-\frac{1}{0.25} \text{ or } - 4 \text{ D.}$$

It is possible to think of the other terms in the lens equation in a similar way. The reciprocal of object and image distances *in metres* gives a dioptric value which is a measure of the vergence of the rays between object or image and the lens. In other words, it is a measure of the degree of convergence or divergence of the rays in question.

The concept of vergence is an important aid to the understanding of the optics of accommodation and presbyopia.

Magnification formulae

Linear magnification

The linear magnification produced by a spherical lens can be calculated from the basic formula:

$$\text{Linear magnification} = \frac{I}{O} = \frac{v}{u}$$

where I is the image size, O is the object size, v is the distance of the image from the principal plane, and u is the distance of the object from the principal plane (Fig. 5.9).

Angular magnification

In ophthalmic practice, actual image and object size are of less importance than the angle subtended at the eye,

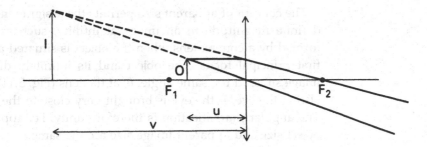

Fig. 5.9 Linear magnification. Convex lens. Object within focal length.

because the angle subtended governs the retinal image size.

Figure 5.10a shows that objects A, B, C and D all subtend angle θ at the eye and produce a retinal image xy. They are all therefore of identical *apparent size*. Apparent size is given by the ratio of object (or image) size divided by its distance from the eye, which is, of course, tan θ. (See Appendix I.) When considering the eye, the angles encountered are small. For small angles the value of tan θ can be taken to be equal to the angles themselves.

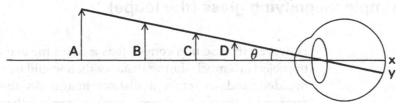

Fig. 5.10a Apparent size: visual angle.

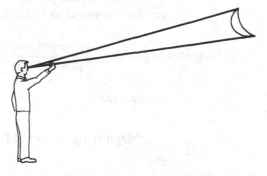

Fig. 5.10b Apparent size: visual angle illustrated. A coin held at arms length obscures the view of the moon.

The concept of apparent size permits the assignment of a definite magnitude to an image at infinity, such as that formed by a convex lens when the object is situated at the first principal focus. The object and its infinitely distant image subtend the same angle, θ, at the lens (Fig. 5.11) and also at the eye, if the eye is brought very close to the lens. The angular magnification is therefore unity, i.e. apparent object size and apparent image size are the same.

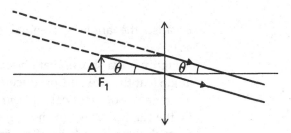

Fig. 5.11 Image formation by convex lens with object at first principal focus: the magnifying glass or loupe.

The simple magnifying glass (the loupe)

However, the use of a convex lens enables the eye to view the object at a much shorter distance than would be possible unaided, and to retain a distinct image. As the object approaches the eye it subtends a greater angle at the eye and the retinal image size increases.

The magnifying power of the lens under these conditions can be expressed as follows:

$$\text{Magnifying power} = \frac{\text{Apparent size of image}}{\text{Apparent size of object}} \text{ at 25 cm from the eye}$$

Alternatively

$$\text{Magnifying power, M,} = \frac{\tan \theta_2}{\tan \theta_1}$$

But

$$\tan \theta_1 = \frac{O}{25}$$

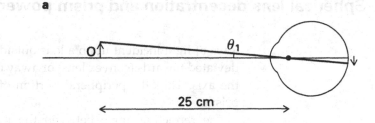

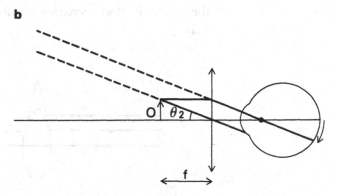

Fig. 5.12 The simple magnifying glass (the loupe). (a) Object viewed at near point of unaided eye, 25 cm, subtends angle θ_1 at the eye. (b) Object viewed close to the eye through a convex lens, with object at first principal focus of convex lens. Object and image subtend angle θ_2 at the eye.

and
$$\tan \theta_2 = \frac{O}{f}$$
thus
$$M = \frac{O}{f} \times \frac{25}{O}$$

$$= \frac{25}{f}$$

But 25 cm $= \frac{1}{4}$ m, and $\frac{1}{f} = F$ dioptres, where F is the power of the lens in dioptres.

Therefore $M = \frac{F}{4}$

Thus, the commonly used $\times 8$ loupe has a lens power of +32 dioptres.

Spherical lens decentration and prism power

Rays of light incident upon a lens outside its axial zone are deviated towards (convex lens) or away from (concave lens) the axis. Thus the peripheral portion of the lens acts as a prism.

The refracting angle between the lens surfaces grows larger as the edge of the lens is approached (Fig. 5.13). Thus the primatic effect increases towards the periphery of the lens.

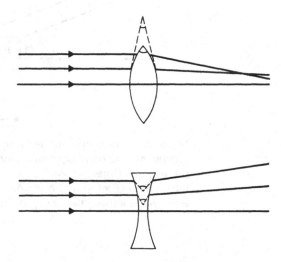

Fig. 5.13 Prismatic deviation by spherical lenses.

Use of a non-axial portion of a lens to gain a prismatic effect is called *decentration* of the lens. Lens decentration is frequently employed in spectacles where a prism is to be incorporated. On the other hand, poor centration of spectacle lenses, especially high power lenses, may produce an unwanted prismatic effect. This is a frequent cause of spectacle intolerance, especially in patients with aphakia or high myopia.

It is thus of importance to be able to predict the prismatic power gained by decentring a spherical lens. This is given by the formula

$$P = F \times D$$

where P is the prismatic power in prism dioptres, F is the lens power in dioptres, and D is the decentration *in centimetres*.

The increasing prismatic power of the more peripheral parts of a spherical lens is the underlying mechanism of spherical aberration (see p. 92). Furthermore, it causes the troublesome ring scotoma and jack-in-the-box effect which give rise to great difficulty to those wearing high-power spectacle lenses (pp. 131, 132).

6   Astigmatic Lenses

All the meridians of each surface of a spherical lens have the same curvature (as parts of a sphere), and refraction is symmetrical about the principal axis.

In an astigmatic lens, all meridians do not have the same curvature, and a point image of a point object cannot be formed. There are two types of astigmatic lenses, namely cylindrical and toric lenses.

Cylindrical lenses

These lenses have one plane surface and the other forms part of a cylinder (Fig. 6.1). Thus, in one meridian the lens has no vergence power and this is called the *axis of the cylinder*. In the meridian at right angles to the axis, the cylinder acts as a spherical lens. The total effect is the

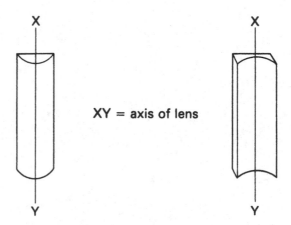

Fig. 6.1   Cylindrical lens.

formation of a line image of a point object. This is called the *focal line*. It is parallel to the axis of the cylinder (Fig. 6.2).

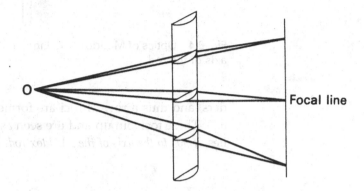

Fig. 6.2 Image formation by convex cylindrical lens of point object, O.

The Maddox rod

This useful device, used in the diagnosis of extraocular muscle imbalance, consists of a series of powerful convex cylindrical lenses mounted side by side in a trial lens (Fig. 6.3).

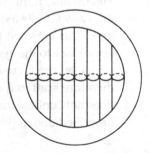

Fig. 6.3 The Maddox rod.

The patient views a distant white point source of light through the Maddox rod, which is placed close to the eye (in the trial frame). The spotlight must be far enough away for its rays to be parallel on reaching the patient (at least 6 m). Light in the meridian parallel to the axis of each cylinder passes through undeviated and *is brought to a focus by the eye* (Fig. 6.4). The Maddox rod consists of a row of such cylin-

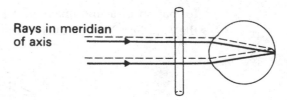

Fig. 6.4 Optics of Maddox rod. Light in the meridian parallel to axis of the rod.

ders, and thus a row of foci are formed on the retina (Fig. 6.5). These foci join up and are seen as a line of light which lies *at 90° to the axis of the Maddox rod.*

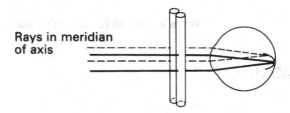

Fig. 6.5 Optics of Maddox rod. To show formation of line of foci by adjacent elements of Maddox rod.

Meanwhile, light incident on the Maddox rod in the meridian at 90° to its axis is converged by each cylinder to a real line focus between the rod and the eye (Fig. 6.6). This focus is too close to the eye for a distinct image to be formed on the retina by the focusing mechanism of the eye. This light is therefore scattered over a wide area of retina (Fig. 6.6) and does not confuse the perception of the composite line image described above (Fig. 6.5).

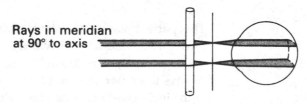

Fig. 6.6 Optics of Maddox rod. Light incident in the meridian at 90° to axis of Maddox rod.

Remember that the line seen by the patient lies at 90° to the axis of the Maddox rod and is formed by the focusing mechanism of the eye. It is not the real line image of the Maddox rod.

The glass of the Maddox rod is tinted red so the composite line image seen by the patient is also red.

Use of the Maddox rod to test muscle balance

To test muscle balance the Maddox rod is placed close in front of the right eye (in the trial frame) and the distant white spotlight is viewed with both eyes. The right eye therefore sees a red line, at 90° to the axis of the Maddox rod, while the left eye sees the white spotlight. Thus the two eyes see dissimilar images and are dissociated, allowing any muscle imbalance to become manifest. To test for horizontal imbalance, the rod must be horizontal to give a vertical line and vice versa. Remember that the eye behind the Maddox rod (conventionally the right) is deviating in the opposite direction to that indicated by the red line (Fig. 6.7).

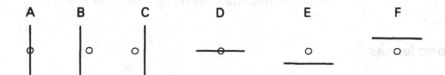

Fig. 6.7 The patient's view (Maddox rod before the right eye).

A	Horizontal orthophoria	
B	Exophoria	The patient has crossed diplopia and this indicates an exophoria ('X'ed diplopia ≡ e̲x̲o̲)
C	Esophoria	
D	Vertical orthophoria	
E	Right hyperphoria	
F	Right hypophoria (= left hyperphoria)	

Any deviation is measured by placing prisms before the left eye until the orthophoric situation is achieved.

Toric surface

Imagine that the cylindrical lens in Fig. 6.1 is picked up by its ends and bent so that the axis XY becomes an arc of a circle. The previously cylindrical surface is now curved in both its vertical and horizontal meridians, but not to the same extent. It is now called a *toric* surface. The meridians of maximum and minimum curvature are called the *principal meridians* and in ophthalmic lenses these are at 90° to each other (Fig. 6.8).

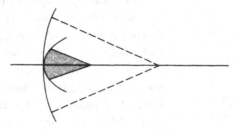

Fig. 6.8 Toric surface. Principal meridians with radii and centres of curvature.

The principal meridian of minimum curvature, and therefore minimum power, is called the *base curve*.

Toric lenses

Lenses with one toric surface are known as toric lenses, or sphero-cylindrical lenses. Such lenses do not produce a single defined image because the principal meridians form separate line foci at right angles to each other.

Between the two line foci the rays of light form a figure known as Sturm's conoid (after the mathematician Sturm who described it in 1838). The distance between the two line foci is called the interval of Sturm (Fig. 6.9). The plane where the two pencils of light intersect is called the circle of least confusion or the circle of least diffusion. Blur circle images only are formed at all other planes lying between F_H and F_V.

A toric lens can be thought of as a spherical lens with a cylindrical lens superimposed upon it. Toric lenses may be defined numerically as a fraction, the spherical power being the numerator and the cylindrical power the denominator.

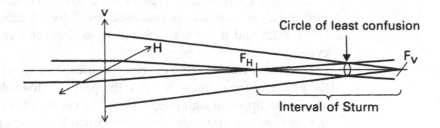

Fig. 6.9 Image formed by toric astigmatic lens – Sturm's conoid.

For example a toric lens with a power of +2 D in one principal meridian and +4 D in the other principal meridian can be regarded as a +2 D sphere with a +2 D cylinder superimposed. This is therefore written as +2.0 DS/+2.0 DC.

Spherical equivalent

It is sometimes useful to calculate the power of the spherical lens of closest overall effect to a given toric lens, known as the spherical equivalent. This reveals whether the eye is essentially hypermetropic, emmetropic or myopic. This consideration is especially important in the choice of intraocular lens power for the individual patient (cf. pp. 134–139).

The *spherical equivalent* power is calculated from the toric lens prescription by algebraic addition of the spherical power and half the cylindrical power, e.g. the spherical equivalent of +2.00 DS/+2.00 DC is +3.00 DS, while that of +2.00 DS/–2.00 DC is +1.00 DS. The focal point of the spherical equivalent would coincide with the circle of least confusion of the toric lens's Sturm's conoid.

The cross-cylinder

In clinical refraction the orientation of the trial cylinder can be checked by superimposing another cylinder with its axis lying obliquely to the axis of the trial cylinder. The power of a cylinder can be checked by superimposing further cylinders of varying power and sign in the same axis as the trial cylinder. These considerations have led to the evolution of the cross-cylinder.

The cross-cylinder is a type of toric lens used during refraction. Its use was popularised by Edward Jackson (1893–1929) and it is often referred to as 'Jackson's cross-cylinder'.

The cross-cylinder is a sphero-cylindrical lens in which the power of the cylinder is twice the power of the sphere and of the opposite sign (Fig. 6.10a). The net result is thus the same as superimposing two cylindrical lenses of equal power but opposite sign with their axes at right angles. The lens is mounted on a handle which is placed at 45° to the axes of the cylinders.

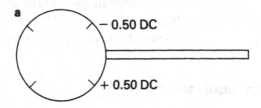

Fig. 6.10a A cross-cylinder. –0.50 DS/+1.0 DC

The axes marked on the lens are the axes of no power of the individual cylinders. The power of each cylinder lies at 90° to the marked axis and coincides with the marked axis (of no power) of the other cylinder (of opposite sign) (Fig. 6.10b).

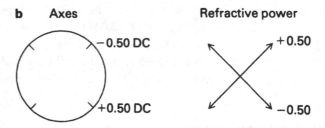

Fig. 6.10b The cross-cylinder showing axes as marked on the lens and refractive power in the principal meridians.

Cross-cylinders are named by the power of the cylinder, and this is marked on the handle. The cross-cylinder illustrated in Figs 6.10a and b would be designated a 1.00 dioptre cross-cylinder. Cross-cylinders are available in two powers, 0.50 and 1.00 dioptre. The 1.00 D cross-cylinder is used to check the axis of the trial cylinder, and the power in patients with poor visual acuity. The 0.50 D cross-cylinder is used to check the power of the trial cylinder where the patient has good vision.

Clinically the cross-cylinder is used to check the axis of the cylinder prescribed and then its power. It can also be used to verify that no cylindrical correction is necessary for the patient if no cylinder was detected on retinoscopy.

In practice the patient is asked to look at the line of test type two lines above the smallest he can see. This is because the cross-cylinder blurs the vision and larger letters are used to make discrimination between the positions of the cross-cylinder easier for the patient.

To check the axis, the cross-cylinder is held before the eye with its handle in line with the axis of the trial cylinder. The cross-cylinder is turned over and the patient asked which position gives a better visual result. The cross-cylinder is held in the preferred position and the axis of the trial cylinder rotated slightly towards the axis of the same sign on the cross-cylinder. The process is repeated until the trial cylinder is in the correct axis for the eye, at which time rotation of the cross-cylinder will offer equally unacceptable visual alterations to the patient.

To check the power of the trial cylinder the cross-cylinder is held with first one axis and then the other overlying the trial cylinder. This has the effect of increasing and then decreasing the power of the trial cylinder.

To confirm the absence of a cylinder, the cross-cylinder is offered as an addition to the trial sphere in four different orientations, with its + axis at 90°, 180°, 45°, and 135°. If the patient prefers one of these options to the sphere alone, a cylindrical correction is necessary. The exact axis and power can then be determined by the methods described above.

To achieve the best results from the test it is important that the patient has the clearest vision possible before the cross-cylinder is used.

7 Optical Prescriptions, Spectacle Lenses

The lenses described in Chapters 5 and 6 have many uses in ophthalmology. Lenses are used as optical aids for patients with refractive errors, in the form of spectacles or contact lenses, and as low vision aids (Chapter 13). Lenses are also an essential component of most of the instruments used in ophthalmology (Chapter 14). In this chapter the use of lenses in spectacles is discussed.

Prescription of lenses

When prescribing a spectacle lens, the properties of the lens required are specified in the following way.

A spherical lens alone is written as, for example, +2.00 DS (dioptre sphere) or –3.25 DS.

In the case of a cylindrical lens alone, both the dioptric power and the orientation of the axis must be specified. The axis of the cylinder is marked on each trial lens by a line, and trial frames are marked according to a standard international convention (Fig. 7.1). Thus, a cylinder of –2.0

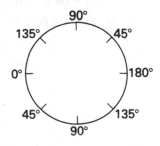

Fig. 7.1 Conventional orientation for cylindrical lenses.

dioptre power, placed with its axis (of no power) vertical is written as −2.0 DC axis 90° (DC = dioptre cylinder).

Often the correction of a refractive error entails the prescription of both a spherical and a cylindrical component, i.e. a toric astigmatic correction. In such a case, at the end of refraction the trial frame contains a spherical lens (e.g. +2.0 DS) and a cylindrical lens (e.g. +1.0 DC axis 90°). The cylindrical lens is usually placed in front of the spherical lens to allow the axis line to be seen.

The prescription is written as +2.00 DS/+1.00 DC axis 90°, and this may be abbreviated to +2.00/+1.00$_{90°}$

Transposition of lenses

When a lens prescription is changed from one lens form to another optically equivalent form, the process is called transposition of the lens.

Simple transposition of spheres

This applies to the alteration of the lens form of spherical lenses. The lens power is given by the algebraic sum of the surface powers (Fig. 7.2).

+1.5 +1.5   0 +3.0 −1.50 +4.50 −6.00 +9.00

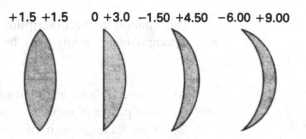

Fig. 7.2   Simple transposition of a +3.0 D spherical lens.

Simple transposition of cylinders

This is a change in the description of a toric astigmatic lens so that the cylinder is expressed in the opposite power. Simple transposition of the cylinder is often necessary when the examiner wishes to compare the present refraction with a previous prescription.

Consider the following example (Fig. 7.3).

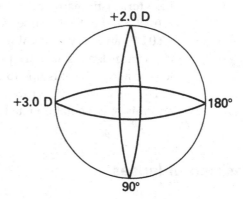

Fig. 7.3 Diagram representing the toric lens

$$\frac{+2.00\ DS}{+1.00\ DC\ \text{axis}\ 90°}$$

showing dioptric power of principal meridia.

The lens depicted in Fig. 7.3 can be described in two ways.

(1) Let the cylindrical element be at axis 90°: the lens is now +2.0 DS/+1.0 DC axis 90°.
(2) Let the cylindrical element be of opposite power and at axis 180°: the lens is now +3.0 DS/–1.0 DC axis 180°.

This change in the description of the lens may be easily accomplished for any lens by performing the following steps.

(a) *Sum.* Algebraic addition of sphere and cylinder gives new power of sphere.
(b) *Sign.* Change sign of cylinder, retaining numerical power.
(c) *Axis.* Rotate axis of cylinder through 90°. (Add 90° if the original axis is at or less than 90°. Subtract 90° from any axis figure greater than 90°.)

Examples   (It is suggested that the reader cover one side of the page to conceal the answers and work through these examples before checking the results.)

$$\frac{+4.0 \text{ DS}}{+1.50 \text{ DC}} \text{ axis } 90° \equiv \frac{+5.50 \text{ DS}}{-1.50 \text{ DC}} \text{ axis } 180°$$

$$\frac{-2.0 \text{ DS}}{-1.0 \text{ DC}} \text{ axis } 170° \equiv \frac{-3.0 \text{ DS}}{+1.0 \text{ DC}} \text{ axis } 80°$$

$$\frac{+1.0 \text{ DS}}{-3.0 \text{ DC}} \text{ axis } 180° \equiv \frac{-2.0 \text{ DS}}{+3.0 \text{ DC}} \text{ axis } 90°$$

$$\frac{-1.50 \text{ DS}}{+2.50 \text{ DC}} \text{ axis } 20° \equiv \frac{+1.0 \text{ DS}}{-2.50 \text{ DC}} \text{ axis } 110°$$

Toric transposition

Toric transposition carries the process one step further and enables a toric astigmatic lens to be exactly defined in terms of its surface powers. A toric astigmatic lens is made with one spherical surface and one toric surface (the latter contributing the cylindrical power). The principal meridian of weaker power of the toric surface is known as the *base curve* of the lens. The base curve must be specified if toric transposition of a lens prescription is required (Fig. 7.4).

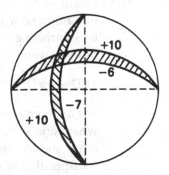

Fig. 7.4 Diagram representing toric astigmatic lens

$$\frac{+4.0 \text{ DS axis } 180°}{-1.0 \text{ DC}}$$

with base curve −6 D.

The toric formula is written in two lines, as a fraction. The top line (numerator) specifies the surface power of the spherical surface. The bottom line (denominator) defines the surface power and axis of the base curve, followed by the surface power and axis of the other principal meridian of the toric surface. For example:

$$\frac{+9.0 \text{ DS}}{-6.0 \text{ DC axis } 90°/-8.0 \text{ DC axis } 180°}$$

The steps of toric transposition are now defined taking the following case as an example.

'Transpose $\dfrac{+3.0 \text{ DS}}{+1.0 \text{ DC axis } 90°}$

to a toric formula to the base curve –6 D.'

(1) Transpose the prescription so that the cylinder and the base curve are of the same sign, for example:

(a) $\dfrac{+3.0 \text{ DS}}{+1.0 \text{ DC axis } 90°}$

becomes

(b) $\dfrac{+4.0 \text{ DS}}{-1.0 \text{ DC axis } 180°}$

(2) Calculate the required power of the spherical surface (the numerator of the final formula). This is obtained by subtracting the base curve power from the spherical power given in (b) in step 1.

+4 D – (–6 D) = +10 D

Put another way, to obtain an overall power of +4.0 D where one surface of the lens has the power –6 D, the other surface must have the power +10 D (cf simple transposition of spheres).

(3) Specify the axis of the base curve. As this is the weaker principal meridian of the toric surface, its axis is at 90° to the axis of the required cylinder found in (b) in step 1. That is:

–6 D axis 90°

(4) Add the required cylinder to the base curve power with its axis as in (b) in step 1

–6 D + (–1 D) = –7 DC axis 180°

The complete toric formula is thus

$$\frac{+10 \text{ DS}}{-6 \text{ DC axis } 90°/-7 \text{ DC axis } 180°}$$

Some further examples for calculation are given below:

Transpose $\dfrac{+4.0 \text{ DS}}{-2.0 \text{ DC axis } 180°} \equiv \dfrac{-4.0 \text{ DS}}{+6.0 \text{ DC axis } 180°/+8.0 \text{ DC axis } 90°}$

to the base curve +6 D

Transpose $\dfrac{-2.0 \text{ DS}}{+3.0 \text{ DC axis } 90°} \equiv \dfrac{+7.0 \text{ DS}}{-6.0 \text{ DC axis } 90°/-9.0 \text{ DC axis } 180°}$

to the base curve −6D

Identification of lenses

In clinical practice it is frequently necessary for the practitioner to identify the type and power of the patient's existing spectacles. This may be done by the following means.

Detection of lens type

It is possible to determine whether a given lens is spherical, astigmatic or a prism by studying the image formed when two lines, crossed at 90°, are viewed through the lens.

Spherical lenses cause no distortion of the cross. However, when the lens is moved from side to side and up and down along the arms of the cross, the cross also appears to move. In the case of a convex lens, the cross appears to move in the opposite direction to the lens, termed as 'against movement', while a movement in the same direction as the lens, a 'with movement', is observed if the lens is concave (Fig. 7.5).

Astigmatic lenses cause distortion of the cross unless their axes coincide with the cross lines. Rotation of the lens thus causes a 'scissors' movement as the crossed lines are progressively displaced (Fig. 7.6). Rotation of a spherical lens has no effect upon the image of the crossed lines.

Once the principal meridians of an astigmatic lens have

a Convex = 'against movement'

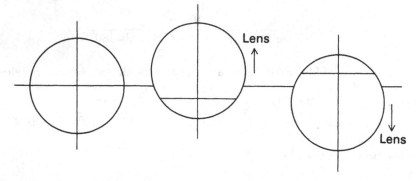

b Concave = 'with movement'

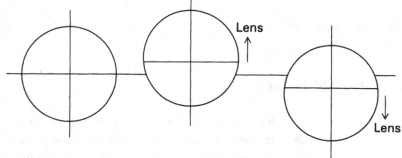

Fig. 7.5 Detection of spherical lenses.

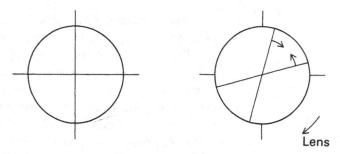

Fig. 7.6 Detection of astigmatic lenses.

been identified, and aligned with the cross, each meridian may be examined as for a spherical lens.

The optical centre of a lens may be found by moving the lens until one cross line is undisplaced. A line is then drawn on the lens surface, superimposed on the undisplaced cross line. The process is then repeated for the cross line at 90°.

The point where the lines drawn on the lens intersect is the optical centre of the lens.

A prism has no optical centre and thus displaces one line of the cross regardless of its position with respect to the cross. Furthermore, the direction of displacement is constant (Fig. 7.7).

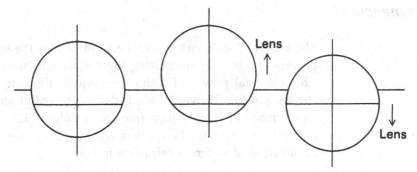

Fig. 7.7   Detection of a prism.

This test is most effective if the cross lines are placed at the furthest convenient distance and the lens held well away from the eye.

Neutralisation of power

The power of a lens can also be found using the technique described above. Once the nature of the unknown lens is determined, lenses of opposite type and known power are superimposed upon the unknown lens until a combination is found which gives no movement of the image of the cross lines when the test is performed. At this point the two lenses are said to 'neutralise' each other, and the dioptric power of the unknown lens must equal that of the trial lens of opposite sign (a + 2.0 D lens neutralises a –2.0 D lens).

In the case of astigmatic lenses, each meridian must be neutralised separately.

Spectacle lenses are named by their back vertex power (see Chapter 9). To measure this accurately, the neutralising lens must be placed in contact with the back surface of the spectacle lens. However, with many highly curved lenses this is not possible and an air space intervenes. It is then better to place the neutralising lens against the front surface of the spectacle lens. Neutralisation is thus somewhat inaccurate for curved lenses of more than about 2 dioptres power and an error of up to 0.50 dioptre may be incurred with powerful lenses. Nevertheless, for relatively low power lenses neutralisation is still a very useful technique.

Lens measure

The Geneva lens measure can be used to find the surface powers of a lens by measuring the surface curvature (Fig. 7.8). The total power of a thin lens equals the sum of its surface powers. However, the instrument is calibrated for lenses made of crown glass (refractive index 1.523) and a correction factor must be applied in the case of lenses made of materials of different refractive indices.

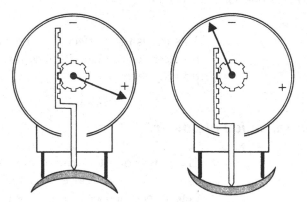

Fig. 7.8 Principle of the Geneva lens measure.

The focimeter

A focimeter is used to measure the vertex power of a lens, the axes and major powers of an astigmatic lens and the power of a prism. It consists of two main parts, a focusing system and an observation system (Fig. 7.9). The focusing system comprises an illuminated target and a collimating lens. A collimating lens is one which renders light parallel. The target is usually a ring of dots formed by a disc in which a circle of small holes is punched and behind which there is

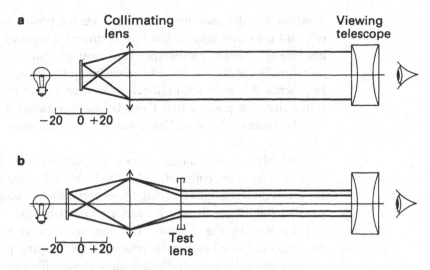

a Collimating lens

Viewing telescope

−20 0 +20

b

−20 0 +20

Test lens

Fig. 7.9 The focimeter.

a light source. Green light is used to eliminate chromatic aberration. The position of the collimating lens is fixed but the target may be moved relative to it. When the target is located at the first principal focus of the collimating lens, the emerging light rays are parallel (Fig. 7.9a). The light emerging from the system is viewed through the observation system which comprises a telescope with an adjustable eyepiece which should be focused at infinity. The eyepiece contains a graticule and a protractor scale for measuring the axes of cylindrical lenses and prismatic power. Before use, the instrument should be set to zero and the eyepiece adjusted until the dots and the graticule are sharply focused. The lens being tested is placed in a special rack which lies at the second principal focus of the collimating lens (Fig. 7.9b)

The focimeter measures the vertex power of the lens surface in contact with the lens rest. When examining spectacle lenses, which are designated by their back vertex power, it is thus important to mount the glasses with the back surface of the lens against the rest. However, when examining a bifocal spectacle lens, as well as measuring the back vertex power of the distance portion, it is necessary to measure the bifocal add, i.e. the extra plus power conferred by the near segment (cf. Chapter 11, Bifocal lenses). Because the supplementary power of the near segment works by reducing the divergence of light from the near object before it enters the distance lens, the front vertex power is the relevant measurement for the near segment. The front vertex power of both the distance and near portions should therefore be measured, the difference being the bifocal add. In practice it is only with bifocals with high power convex (plus) distance powers that there is any significant difference between the front and back vertex power measurement of the bifocal add.

Movement of the target allows the vergence of light emerging from the collimating lens to be varied. The target is moved until the light entering the observation telescope is parallel (Fig. 7.9b) in which case a focused image of the target is seen by the observer. The distance through which the target is moved is directly related to the dioptric power of the lens under test. The instrument is so calibrated that the power of the lens can be read off in dioptres.

The image of the target is seen as a ring of dots when a spherical lens is tested. However, in the case of an astigmatic lens the target must be focused separately for the two principal meridians. The dots of the target are then seen as drawn out lines, the length of the lines being proportional to the difference between the two principal powers, that is, the cylindrical power of the lens under test.

To examine an astigmatic lens on the focimeter, e.g. the lens shown in Fig. 7.10a, the instrument is adjusted until one set of line foci is in focus (Fig. 7.10a(i)) and the reading (+1.0 D) recorded. The instrument is further adjusted until

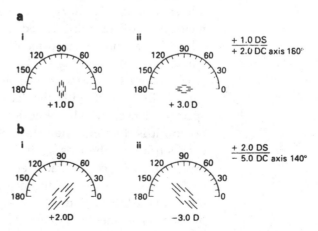

Fig. 7.10 Use of the focimeter to diagnose astigmatic lenses. Image seen.

the second set of line foci come into focus (Fig. 7.10a(ii)) and the reading (+3.0 D) and axis (180°) of the lines recorded. The first reading gives the spherical power of the lens. The cylindrical power is calculated by algebraic subtraction of the first reading from the second (+3) – (+1) = +2 D. The axis of the cylinder corresponds to the axis of the second reading, i.e. 180°. Figure 7.10b shows another example.

A spectacle lens may have a prismatic effect either because it has a prism incorporated in it or because it has been decentred. If there is a prism incorporated in the lens, it will be impossible to bring the image of the target to the centre of the eyepiece graticule. The cross-lines of the graticule are calibrated in intervals of one prism dioptre enabling the prism power to be determined. The image is seen displaced towards the base of the prism because the image of the target is inverted by the eyepiece telescope.

In order to detect the prismatic effect of a lens which has been decentred, the centre of the lens should be marked (most machines incorporate a marker). The marked spectacles are then put on to the patient and the degree of decentration of the lens measured by observing the relationship between the centre of the patient's pupil and the optical centre of the lens. Prism power is given by the equation

$$P = F \times D$$

where P is the prismatic power in prism dioptres, F is the lens power in dioptres, and D is the decentration in *centimetres*.

Automated focimeter

The degree to which a beam of light is deflected as it passes through a lens depends on the focal and prismatic power of the lens and the distance from its optical centre. This is the principle on which an automatic focimeter is based. A square pattern of four parallel beams of light is passed through the lens to be tested. The deflected beams strike a photosensitive surface which measures the deviation of each of the beams from its original path to compute the lens measurements.

Tinted lenses

A tinted lens modifies the spectral profile of the radiation passing through it. Tints are either absorptive or reflective; absorptive tints absorb light passing through them, whereas a reflective tint reflects unwanted wavelengths. Unequal absorption of different wavelengths produces a coloured tint. For example, a yellow-tinted filter absorbs all wavelengths of light except those in the yellow part of the spectrum, which it transmits. A neutral density filter absorbs all wavelengths to the same degree and does not alter the spectral composition of the light. Tints may be of fixed colour (cf. fluorescein angiography) or photochromic (in which transmission characteristics vary with the intensity of incident light). The purpose of tinted lenses may be to screen out unwanted or harmful radiation (e.g. laser protective goggles) or cosmetic.

A tint may be added to a lens by permeation, by means of a coating or as a solid tint. Most plastic lenses are tinted by immersion in a dye which permeates the lens to a uniform depth to produce an even tint; darker tints are produced by prolonged immersion. Coating applied to the lens surface may be absorptive (Cr, NiCr, MgF_2, SiO) or reflective (Cr, NiCr). A solid tint is incorporated evenly throughout the lens and absorption of radiation is therefore greater where the lens is thicker. The performance of a tinted lens is described by a transmittance curve which plots the percentage transmission of incident light for each wavelength.

Ultraviolet filters

Ultraviolet light comprises approximately 5% of total solar radiation. Ozone in the earth's atmosphere absorbs almost all solar UV-C radiation. Of the remainder which strikes the earth's surface, approximately 90% is UV-A and 10% is UV-B (cf. electromagnetic spectrum, Chapter 1). Ultraviolet light exposure may also come from arc welding and UV-emitting light bulbs. CR39 lenses absorb UV light shorter than 370 nm.

Infrared (IR) wavelengths near 1400 nm are very hazardous; filters for these wavelengths are usually incorporated into protective goggles and face masks. Heat absorbing filters also act as IR filters but maximise the transmission of visible light.

Blue light filters vary in tint between yellow and red. They increase contrast and facilitate distinction of light and dark areas and are used by mountaineers and skiers.

Photochromic lenses

A photochromic lens changes its transmission characteristics depending upon the intensity of incident radiation. The lens becomes darker in brighter light. The process of darkening is more rapid than that of lightening. The reactions in glass and plastic are different.

Glass photochromic lenses comprise colourless silver halide crystals suspended in borosilicate. Electromagnetic energy dissociates the silver and halogen to cause darkening. Each type of glass has an optimum activating (usually UV or blue) and bleaching wavelength; the tint will depend upon which wavelength predominates. Heat opposes the effect of light. Thus, glass darkens more easily when cold and lightens more easily when warm. A glass lens becomes gradually darker over time if it is used repeatedly.

A number of organic photochromic compounds are used to coat or impregnate plastic lenses. They are more wavelength specific and undergo structural transformation when stimulated. Fatiguability of the material over time reduces the darkening which occurs. The time delay in the reaction of photochromic lenses makes them unsuitable for use where lighting conditions change rapidly, e.g. when driving through tunnels.

Anti-reflective coatings

The reflection of light from the surface of a lens may be reduced by coating it with a material the thickness of which is a quarter of the wavelength of the incident light (Fig. 7.11). Light rays which are reflected from the surface of the lens travel a distance of one half of a wavelength further

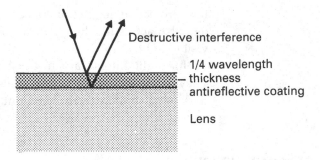

Fig. 7.11 Antireflective coating.

than those which are reflected from the surface of the anti-reflective coating. This causes destructive interference and reduces the reflection of light (cf. Interference, Chapter 1).

In contrast, a coating which has a thickness half the wavelength of the incident light produces a mirror coating because of constructive interference. Any wavelength may be selectively reflected by a coating which is half a wavelength thick. Mirror coatings are usually combined with an absorptive tint.

8　Aberrations of Optical Systems Including the Eye*

In practice, the images formed by the various refracting surfaces or systems described in previous chapters fall short of theoretical perfection. Imperfections of image formation are due to several mechanisms, or aberrations, and these have been analysed and means devised to reduce or eliminate their effect. The refracting system of the eye is also subject to aberrations, but there are correcting mechanisms built into the eye itself.

Chromatic aberration

When white light is refracted at an optical interface, it is dispersed into its component wavelengths or colours (see Dispersion, Chapter 3, pp. 40, 42. Fig. 3.12). The shorter the wavelength of the light, the more it is deviated on refraction. Thus a series of coloured images are formed when white light is incident upon a spherical lens (Fig. 8.1).

When lenses are used in instruments, it is desirable to eliminate chromatic aberration.

Correction of chromatic aberration

Achromatic lens systems

The dispersive power (Chapter 3, pp. 40–42) of a material is independent of its refractive index. Thus, there are materials

---

*The form of the reduced eye (Chapter 9) is used in the diagrams in this chapter.

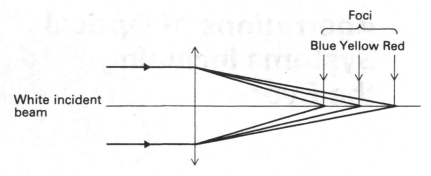

Fig. 8.1 Chromatic aberration.

of high dispersive power but low refractive index, and vice versa.

Achromatic lens systems are composed of elements (lenses) of varying material combined so that the dispersion is neutralised while the overall refractive power is preserved. (For example, by combining a convex lens of high refractive power and low dispersive power with a concave lens of low refractive power but higher dispersive power, the aberration can be neutralised while preserving most of the convex lens refractive power.) The earliest achromatic lenses were made by combining elements of flint and crown glass.

Ocular chromatic aberration

Refraction by the human eye is also subject to chromatic aberration, the total dispersion from the red to the blue image being approximately 2.00 D. The emmetropic eye focuses for the yellow–green (555 nm) as this is the peak wavelength of the photopic relative luminosity curve. This wavelength focus lies between the blue and red foci, being slightly nearer to the red (Fig. 8.2).

Duochrome test

In clinical practice the chromatic aberration of the eye is made use of in the duochrome test. The test consists of two ranks of black Snellen letters, silhouetted against illuminated coloured glass. The upper rank is mounted on red

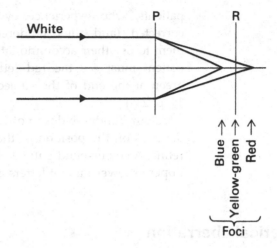

Fig. 8.2 Chromatic aberration, emmetropic eye. P = principal plane, R = retina.

glass, and the lower rank is on green glass. Red and green are used because their wavelength foci straddle the yellow–green by equal amounts (approximately 0.40 D on either side). The patient views the letters by means of red and green light respectively, and can easily tell which appear clearer. The test is sensitive to an alteration in refraction of 0.25 D or less. A myopic eye sees the red letters more clearly than the green (Fig. 8.3) while a hypermetropic eye sees the green letters more distinctly (cf Chapter 10 for definitions of myopia and hypermetropia).

The test is of particular use in the refraction of myopic

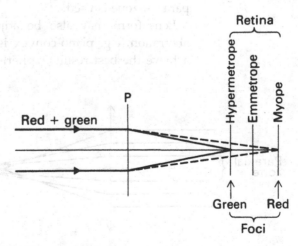

Fig. 8.3 Duochrome test.

patients, who experience eye strain if they are over-corrected (and thus rendered hypermetropic), forcing them to use their accommodation for distance vision. The patient must see the red letters more clearly than the green at the end of the subjective refraction (cf. Chapter 14, p. 236).

Colour blindness does not invalidate the test because it depends on the position of the image with respect to the retina. A colour-blind patient should be asked whether the upper or lower rank of letters appears clearer.

Spherical aberration

In Chapter 5 the prismatic effect of the peripheral parts of spherical lenses was discussed (Fig. 5.13 and text). It was seen that the prismatic effect of a spherical lens is least in the paraxial zone and increases towards the periphery of the lens. Thus, rays passing through the periphery of the lens are deviated more than those passing through the paraxial zone of the lens (Fig. 8.4).

Correction of spherical aberration

Spherical aberration may be reduced by occluding the periphery of the lens by the use of 'stops' so that only the paraxial zone is used.

Lens form may also be adjusted to reduce spherical aberration, e.g. plano-convex is better than biconvex. To achieve the best results, spherical surfaces must be aban-

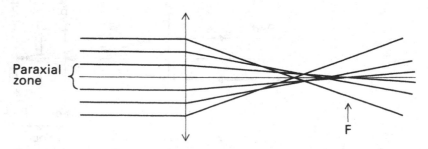

Fig. 8.4 Spherical aberration.

doned and the lenses ground with *aplanatic surfaces*, that is, the peripheral curvature is less than the central curvature (Fig. 8.5).

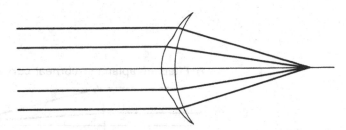

Fig. 8.5 Aplanatic (aspheric) curve to correct spherical aberration.

Another technique of reducing spherical aberration is to employ a doublet. This consists of a principal lens and a somewhat weaker lens of different refractive index cemented together (Fig. 8.6). The weaker lens must be of opposite power, and because it too has spherical aberration, it will reduce the power of the periphery of the principal lens more than the central zone. Usually, such doublets are designed to be both aspheric and achromatic.

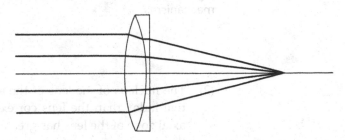

Fig. 8.6 Diagram showing the principle of the aspheric doublet lens.

Ocular spherical aberration

The effect of spherical aberration in the human eye is reduced by several factors (Fig. 8.7).

(1)   The anterior corneal surface is flatter peripherally than at its centre, and therefore acts as an aplanatic surface.

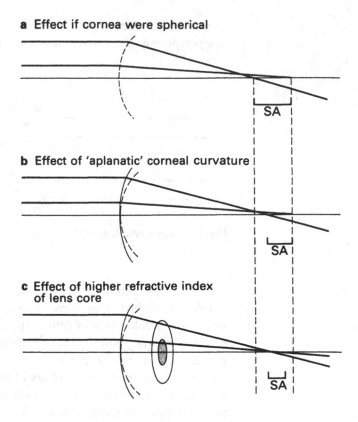

Fig. 8.7 Ocular spherical aberration (SA): compensatory mechanisms.

(2) The nucleus of the lens of the eye has a higher refractive index than the lens cortex (Chapter 9). Thus the axial zone of the lens has greater refractive power than the periphery.

(3) Furthermore, in the eye the iris acts as a stop to reduce spherical aberration. The impairment of visual acuity that occurs when the pupil is dilated is almost entirely due to spherical aberration. Optimum pupil size is 2–2.5 mm.

(4) Finally, the retinal cones are much more sensitive to light which enters the eye paraxially than to light which enters obliquely through the peripheral cornea (Stiles–Crawford effect). This directional sensitivity of the cone photoreceptors limits the visual effects of the residual spherical aberration in the eye.

Oblique astigmatism

Oblique astigmatism is an aberration which occurs when rays of light traverse a spherical lens obliquely. When a pencil of light strikes the lens surfaces obliquely a toric effect is introduced. The emerging rays form a Sturm's conoid with two line foci (Fig. 8.8).

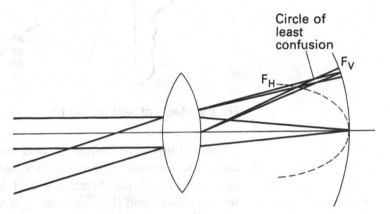

Fig. 8.8 Oblique astigmatism. F_H and F_V represent the horizontal and vertical line foci of a Sturm's conoid.

Oblique astigmatism occurs with spectacle lenses when the line of sight is not parallel with the principal axis of the lens. This is unavoidable in the case of the near portion of a multifocal lens (p. 144). It may also be a cause of reduced acuity in patients with restricted eye movement who adopt a compensatory head posture and look obliquely through peripheral portions of their spectacle lenses. Obviously, the higher the spectacle lens power, the greater the unwanted cylindrical power induced by the aberration.

In daily life adults spend most time looking slightly downward from the primary position, and spectacles are therefore made with the lower borders of the lenses tilted towards the cheek (pantoscopic tilt, Fig. 8.9). This also slightly reduces the obliquity of the reading portion of multifocal lenses (p. 144). However, it may be a cause of intolerance in high power spectacle wearers if new frames are dispensed which have a different angle of pantoscopic tilt from the patient's previous glasses.

Furthermore, oblique astigmatism is considerably affected by the form of the lens used. It is much worse in biconvex and biconcave lenses than in meniscus lenses.

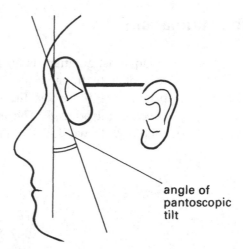

angle of
pantoscopic
tilt

Fig. 8.9 Angle of pantoscopic tilt.

Calculations have been made and tables compiled indicating the optimum form of single lenses for reducing both spherical and oblique aberrations. Such lenses are known as *best form lenses*, and they are usually in meniscus form.

Ocular oblique astigmatism

This aberration occurs in the human eye but its visual effect is minimal. The factors which reduce ocular oblique astigmatism are as follows:

(1) The aplanatic curvature of the cornea reduces oblique astigmatism as well as spherical aberration.
(2) The retina is not a plane surface, but a spherical surface. In practice the radius of curvature of the retina in the emmetropic eye means that the circle of least confusion of the Sturm's conoid formed by oblique astigmatism (Fig. 8.8) falls on the retina.
(3) Finally, the astigmatic image falls on peripheral retina which has relatively poor resolving power compared with the retina at the macula. Visual appreciation of the astigmatic image is therefore limited.

Coma

Coma is really spherical aberration applied to light coming from points not lying on the principal axis. Rays passing through the periphery of the lens are deviated more than the central rays and come to a focus nearer the principal axis (Fig. 8.10). This results in unequal magnification of the image formed by different zones of the lens. The composite image is not circular but elongated like a coma or comet.

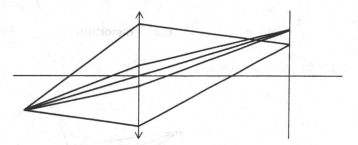

Fig. 8.10 Coma aberration.

Correction of coma aberration

As in the case of oblique astigmatism this aberration can be avoided by limiting rays to the axial area of the lens, and by using the principal axis of the lens rather than a subsidiary axis.

Ocular coma aberration is not of practical importance for the reasons given under oblique astigmatism.

Image distortion

When an extended object is viewed through a spherical lens, the edges of the object, viewed through the peripheral zones of the lens, are distorted (Fig. 8.11). This is due to the increased prismatic effect of the periphery of the lens which produces uneven magnification of the object. A concave lens causes 'barrel' distortion while a convex lens causes 'pincushion' distortion. These effects prove a real nuisance to wearers of high-power spectacle lenses, e.g. aphakic patients.

Curvature of field

The term 'curvature of field' indicates that a plane object gives rise to a curved image (Fig. 8.12). This occurs even

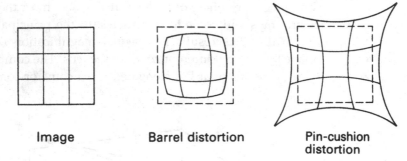

Image   Barrel distortion   Pin-cushion
                                           distortion

Fig. 8.11   Image distortion.

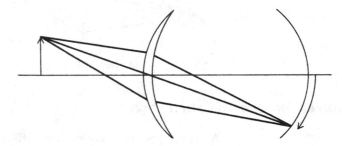

Fig. 8.12   Curvature of field.

when spherical aberration, oblique astigmatism and coma
have been eliminated. The effect is dependent upon the
refractive index of the lens material and the curvature of the
lens surfaces.

Ocular curvature of field

In the eye the curvature of the retina compensates for curvature of field.

9   Refraction by the Eye

The thin lens formula (Chapter 5) is inadequate to deal with the refracting system of the eye, which is composed of a number of refracting surfaces separated by relatively long distances.

The theory and formula of refraction by thick lenses can be directly applied to the eye. Refraction by thick lenses is therefore considered below, and the principles subsequently applied to the eye.

Thick lens theory

Cardinal points

It will be recalled that the thin lens formula ignores lens thickness and considers refraction only at the two lens surfaces (Chapter 5). For a thick lens this approach is invalidated by the greater separation of the two refracting surfaces by the lens substance. The full mathematical analysis of refraction by a thick lens is very complex. It has been simplified by the introduction of the concept of *principal points* and *principal planes*. These are hypothetical planes and points such that a ray incident at the first principal point or plane, P_1, leaves the second principal point or plane, P_2, at the same vertical distance from the principal axis (Fig. 9.1). The exact position of the principal point is calculated from the curvatures of the lens surfaces, the lens thickness and the refractive index of the lens material. The principal planes intersect the principal axis at right angles at the principal points.

There are two further points, the *nodal points*, N_1 and N_2, which correspond to the centre of a thin lens. Any ray

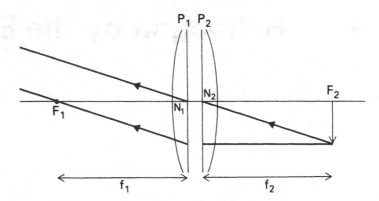

Fig. 9.1 Thick lens. Cardinal points.

directed towards the first nodal point, N_1, leaves the lens as if from the second nodal point, N_2, and parallel with its original direction, i.e. undeviated. When the medium on both sides of the thick lens is the same, the nodal points coincide with the principal points. When the media on opposite sides of the lens are different, the nodal points do not coincide with the principal points.

The *principal foci*, F_1 and F_2, have the same meaning as for a thin lens (Chapter 5), the focal lengths, f_1 and f_2, being measured from the principal points (see below).

Vertex and equivalent power of thick lenses.

Figures 9.1 and 9.2 show that the principal points do not lie on the surface of the lens. They may lie within the lens or, in meniscus form lenses, outside the lens substance. In practice, the measurement given by instruments such as the focimeter is the distance of the principal focus from the central surface or vertex of the lens. This distance is the anterior or posterior *vertex focal length*, AVFL or PVFL, and it must be distinguished from the focal length, f_1 or f_2. Furthermore note that the anterior and posterior vertex focal lengths are not equal to each other (Fig. 9.2).

The reciprocal of the posterior vertex focal length, expressed in metres, is the posterior *vertex power*, expressed in dioptres. An alternative term is the *back vertex power*. This value differs from the 'true' focal power or *equivalent power* of the lens. The *equivalent power* of a thick lens is calculated

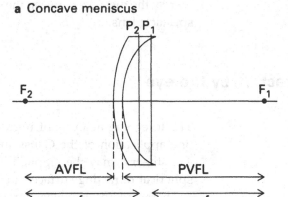

a Concave meniscus

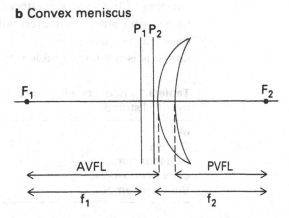

b Convex meniscus

Fig. 9.2   Thick lens: true and vertex focal lengths.

from the two surface powers plus a correction for vergence change due to lens thickness. The discrepancy between equivalent and back vertex power may be a cause of error in dispensing high-powered spectacle lenses, or highly curved contact lenses. However, lens manufacturers and dispensing opticians are aware of this problem, and mathematical tables exist which allow the appropriate adjustment to be made.

Spectacle lenses are graded by their back vertex power as it is their posterior vertex focal length which is relevant to the correction of optical defects in the eye. The second principal focus of the lens must correspond to the far point of the eye if a clear retinal image is to be formed. This is fully explained and illustrated in Chapter 10. Back vertex power should not be confused with back vertex distance, which is merely the distance between the eye and the back vertex of a spectacle lens.

Refraction by the eye

The foregoing analysis of refraction by a thick lens is just one application of the Gaussian theory of cardinal points. The theory may be applied to any system of coaxial spherical refracting surfaces, including the human eye.

There are three major refracting interfaces to be considered in the eye, the anterior corneal surface and the two surfaces of the lens. The effect of the posterior corneal surface is very small compared with these three as the difference in refractive index between corneal stroma and aqueous is not large (Table 9.1).

Table 9.1 Refractive indices of the transparent media of the eye (Gullstrand).

(Air	1.000)
Cornea	1.376
Aqueous humour	1.336
Lens (cortex-core)	1.386–1.406
Vitreous humour	1.336

In order to calculate the cardinal points, the radii of curvature, and distances separating the refracting surfaces must also be known. These have been determined experimentally by several observers. As in the case of any anatomical measurement there is some physiological variation and the values given are the means. The results of Gullstrand are given here (Tables 9.1, 9.2, 9.3) as it is on these

Table 9.2 Position of refracting surfaces of the eye (in mm behind anterior corneal surface) (Gullstrand).

Cornea, anterior surface	0
Cornea, posterior surface	0.5
Lens, anterior surface	3.6
Lens, posterior surface	7.2
Lens core, anterior surface	4.146*
Lens core, posterior surface	6.565*

* Calculated values

Table 9.3 Radii of curvature of refracting surfaces of the eye (in mm) (Gullstrand).

Cornea, anterior surface	7.7
Cornea, posterior surface	6.8
Lens, anterior surface	10.0
Lens, posterior surface	−6.0
Lens core, anterior surface	7.911*
Lens core, posterior surface	−5.76*

* Calculated values

that the given calculations of the schematic and reduced eye are based. These measurements are known as the *optical constants* of the eye. However, there are several other sets of measurements available from other observers which differ slightly one from another. No one set is in general standard use.

The schematic eye

In the schematic eye, as described by Gullstrand, the refracting system is expressed in terms of its cardinal points (measured in mm behind the anterior corneal surface; Table 9.4).

Table 9.4 Schematic eye, cardinal points (distance in mm behind anterior corneal surface) (Gullstrand).

First principal point P_1	1.35
Second principal point P_2	1.60
First nodal point N_1	7.08*
Second nodal point N_2	7.33*
First focal point	−15.7
Second focal point	24.4
Refractive power	+58.64 D

* Calculated by Percival (1928).

Note that the nodal points, via which rays of light pass undeviated (p. 54), are removed from the principal points, which lie at the intersection of the principal planes with the principal axis (Fig. 9.3). This is because the refracting media on each side of the refracting system of the eye are different, namely air ($n = 1$) and vitreous ($n = 1.336$).

The nodal points straddle the posterior pole of the crys-

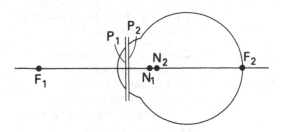

Fig. 9.3 The schematic eye.

talline lens. The pupil of the eye allows only a relatively small paraxial pencil of light to enter the eye. Such paraxial rays are refracted and concentrated through the nodal points and adjacent posterior lens substance. Therefore even a small posterior polar cataract produces gross impairment of vision when the pupil is small.

The reduced eye

Matters were simplified further by Listing (1853) who chose a single principal point lying midway between the two principal points of the schematic eye. A single nodal point was postulated in the same way, and the focal lengths adjusted with reference to the new principal point. The result is the *reduced eye* (Fig. 9.4, Table 9.5), in which the eye is treated as a single refracting surface of power +58.6 D.

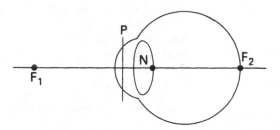

Fig. 9.4 The reduced eye.

Many sets of figures exist for the reduced eye. Those quoted here are based on Gullstrand's data (Duke-Elder, *System of Ophthalmology*, Vol. V, p. 121).

It must be emphasised that the distances given for the focal points are measured from the anterior corneal surface.

Table 9.5 The reduced eye (distances in mm behind anterior corneal surface) (after Gullstrand).

Principal point P	1.35
Nodal point N	7.08
First focal point	−15.7
Second focal point	24.13

The corresponding focal lengths, measured from the principal point, are −17.05 mm and 22.78 mm.

Note that the nodal point lies in the posterior part of the lens, while the second focal point lies 24.13 mm behind the cornea, i.e. on the retina of the normal eye.

The anterior focal length of the aphakic eye was found experimentally to be −23.23 mm (the first focal point lying 21.88 mm in front of the cornea). This gives a calculated power of +43 D for the aphakic eye. The crystalline lens thus has an effective power *in situ* of +15 D (the difference between the power of the phakic and aphakic eye [58 D − 43 D]). Its actual power, taken in isolation from the other refractive elements of the eye, is given by Gullstrand as +19 D. The discrepancy results from the fact that *in vivo* the lens is only one element in a larger refracting system.

The cornea is the only refracting element remaining in the aphakic eye. From the above figures it thus has a power of 43 D, three times as powerful as the crystalline lens in the intact eye. The relatively greater power of the cornea is due to the greater difference in refractive index between air (1.000) and cornea (1.376), as compared with aqueous and vitreous humour (1.336) and lens (1.406), i.e. a difference of 0.376 as opposed to 0.140 (0.070 × 2 because both the anterior and the posterior lens surfaces contribute to the power of the crystalline lens).

A dramatic example of the importance of the air/cornea interface occurs when a swimmer opens his eyes under water. He finds his vision is blurred. The difference in refractive index between water and cornea is only 0.040 (i.e. cornea 1.376 − water 1.336). This problem is eliminated by the swimmer keeping air in front of the cornea by wearing goggles.

The form of the reduced eye is used in all the subsequent discussion of the optics of the eye. The student is advised to commit the values to memory.

Reduced eye – construction of retinal image

Using the reduced eye, it is simple to construct the retinal image formed under various conditions (see Chapter 10).

The reduced eye itself is represented by two parallel lines, which indicate the principal plane, P, and the retina, R. These intersect the principal axis (optical axis) at right angles. The nodal point, N, is indicated by a point, as is the anterior focus, F_a. The second principal focus, F_2, falls on the retina in the emmetropic eye (Fig. 9.5).

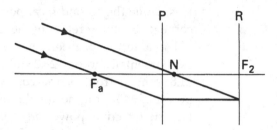

Fig. 9.5 Reduced eye – image formation.

Two rays are used to construct the image formed by parallel light incident upon the eye:

(1) A ray passing through the anterior focus, F_a, which after refraction at the principal plane, P, continues parallel to the principal axis.
(2) A ray passing through the nodal point, N, undeviated.

The size of the retinal image may also be calculated from the same construction. It can be seen from Fig. 9.6 that the light subtends angle α at the nodal point, N, as well as at the anterior focus, F_a. *Retinal image size is therefore directly related to the angle subtended by an object at the nodal point (f_1 being*

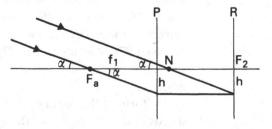

Fig. 9.6 Reduced eye – retinal image size.

constant in the individual eye). Because tan $\alpha = h/f_1$, the retinal image size $h = \tan \alpha \times f_1$. The angle α subtended by an object at the nodal point is called the *visual angle* (Figs 9.6 and 9.7).

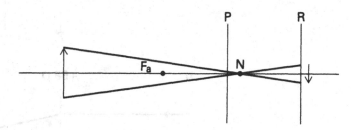

Fig. 9.7 Visual angle – near object.

It will be appreciated that, as an object of given size approaches the eye, it subtends a greater visual angle and thus appears larger (cf. the loupe, Chapter 5).

Variable states of emmetropia

In the emmetropic eye, the second principal focus falls on the retina. Parallel incident light is therefore focused on the retina, without accommodative effort.

The emmetropic state is compatible with a range of refractive powers, if the axial length of the eye is appropriate to its dioptric power (Fig. 9.8).

Accommodation of the eye

If the refractive power of an emmetropic eye were fixed and unalterable, only objects at infinity would be clearly seen. Light from nearer objects would be brought to a focus beyond the second principal focus, F_2 (see convex lenses, Chapter 5), and no clear image would be formed on the retina.

This problem is overcome by the ability of the eye to increase its dioptric power. The crystalline lens is held suspended under tension by the suspensory ligament which attaches it to the ring of ciliary muscle. Ciliary muscle contraction reduces the tension on the suspensory ligament

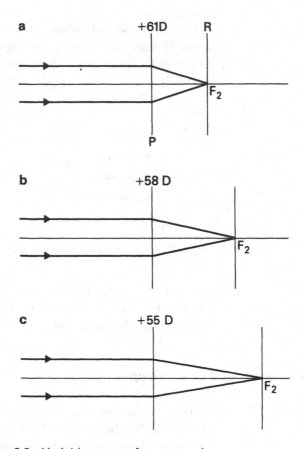

Fig. 9.8   Variable states of emmetropia.

and lens, allowing the lens to assume a more globular shape (Fig. 9.9). The curvatures of the lens surfaces and the lens thickness are increased and thus the dioptric power is increased. Most of the change in curvature occurs at the anterior lens surface, which moves forwards slightly

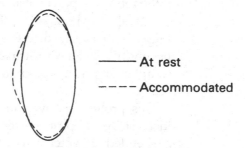

Fig. 9.9   Accommodation. Diagram illustrating change in crystalline lens form.

towards the cornea. This ability of the eye to increase its dioptric power is called *accommodation*.

Before analysing the process of accommodation further it is necessary to define certain terms:

(1)   The *far point* of distinct vision is the position of an object such that its image falls on the retina in the relaxed eye, i.e. in the absence of accommodation. The far point of the emmetropic eye is at infinity.

(2)   The *near point* of distinct vision is the nearest point at which an object can be clearly seen when maximum accommodation is used.

(3)   The *range of accommodation* is the distance between the far point and the near point.

(4)   The *amplitude of accommodation* is the difference in dioptric power between the eye at rest and the fully accommodated eye.

(5)   The dioptric power of the resting eye is called its *static* refraction.

(6)   The dioptric power of the accommodated eye is called its *dynamic* refraction.

Mathematically, the amplitude of accommodation can be calculated from the reciprocals of the near and far point distances measured in metres. These are the *dioptric values* of the near and far point distances. The amplitude of accommodation is given by the formula

$$A = P - R$$

where A is the amplitude of accommodation in dioptres; P is the dioptric value of the near point distance; and R is the dioptric value of the far point distance.

Applying this formula to the case of an emmetropic eye with a near point of 10 cm,

$$P = 10\,D \text{ (the reciprocal of 0.1 m)}$$
$$R = 0 \text{ (the reciprocal of infinity is zero)}$$
therefore $A = 10\,D$.

To calculate the accommodative power required to focus an intermediate point within the range of accommodation the formula is amended to

$$A = V - R$$

where A is the accommodative power required, in dioptres; V is the dioptric value of the intermediate point; R is the dioptric value of the far point (the far point distance in hypermetropia, being behind the eye, carries a negative sign).

Thus, to focus an object at 1 m, the emmetropic eye must exert one dioptre of accommodative power ($A = 1 - 0$).

The amplitude of accommodation declines with advancing age, giving rise to the condition of presbyopia, the inability to focus near objects. This requires spectacle correction and will be discussed later (Chapter 10).

Accommodative convergence/accommodation ratio

In order to view a near object, the eyes must not only accommodate to ensure clear retinal images, but they must also converge to maintain binocular single vision. The two functions are strongly linked and the number of prism dioptres of convergence which accompanies each dioptre of accommodation, the accommodative convergence/accommodation ratio (AC/A) ratio, is relatively constant for each individual. The normal range for the AC/A ratio is 3:1 to 5:1.

The AC/A ratio may be measured by various methods, one of the more accurate being the heterophoria method. This measures the ocular deviation for distance and near with full spectacle correction:

$$AC/A = IPD + (D_d - D_n)/D$$

where IPD is the interpupillary distance in cm, D_n is the ocular deviation for near, D_d is the ocular deviation for distance and D is the near fixation distance in dioptres. (By convention a positive (+) value denotes an esodeviation and a negative (−) value an exodeviation.)

The ratio may also be measured by the gradient method which uses a minus lens rather than a near object to stimulate accommodation. The calculated values are less than and possibly more accurate than those calculated by the heterophoria method:

$$AC/A = (D_d - D_n)/D$$

where D is the power of the minus lens used to induce accommodation.

In clinical practice, an abnormally high AC/A ratio is betrayed by a much larger angle of esotropia for near than for distance. If the AC/A ratio is abnormally high, the condition of convergence excess esotropia may result, in which the eyes are straight for distance but break down to a convergent squint for near. It is important to distinguish this condition from esotropia that is similar for near and distance because the optical and surgical managements differ. Convergence excess esotropia may be controlled with bifocal spectacles, the distance portion incorporating the full hypermetropic distance correction and the near portion having further plus power so that little or no accommodation is required for near, and binocular near vision is facilitated.

If surgery is appropriate, recession of both medial recti is effective in convergence excess esotropia whereas recession of one medial rectus with resection of the ipsilateral lateral rectus is more effective in esotropia without convergence excess.

Catoptric images

Information regarding the changes in lens form during accommodation has come from studies of the catoptric images of the eye.

The changes occurring in the lens during accommodation are inaccessible to direct measurement, and therefore an indirect method must be employed. Similarly the optical constants of the eye (Tables 9.1–9.3) must also be measured indirectly.

Each refracting interface in the eye also acts as a spherical mirror, reflecting a small portion of the light incident upon it (Chapter 2). Four images are therefore formed by reflection at the four interfaces, the anterior and posterior corneal surfaces and the anterior and posterior lens surfaces. These images are called *catoptric images* or *Purkinje–Sanson images* (Fig. 9.10). The latter name honours Purkinje who first described them and Sanson who first used them for diagnostic purposes.

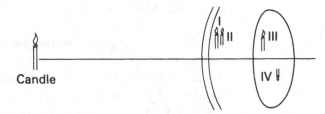

Fig. 9.10   Purkinje–Sanson images. Apparent positions as seen by the observer.

Images I, II and III (from anterior corneal, posterior corneal and anterior lens surfaces respectively) are erect, virtual images because they are formed by convex reflecting surfaces (see Chapter 2).

Image IV (from the posterior lens surface) is a real, inverted image because it is formed by a concave reflecting surface (see Chapter 2).

When using images II, III and IV to make measurements, account must be taken of refraction of the reflected light as it re-emerges from the eye (cf. real and apparent depth, Chapter 3). Figure 9.10 shows the apparent positions of the images when viewed by the observer. However, the actual images lie deeper in the eye: image I lies just behind the anterior lens capsule, and image II is close behind it. Image III is located in the vitreous, and image IV, as it comes from the concave posterior lens surface, is inverted and in the anterior lens substance.

Use of the first image (image I) to study the anterior corneal curvature is routine in clinical practice. The regularity of the curvature is examined using Placido's disc, and the radius of curvature is measured using the keratometer. These instruments are described in Chapter 14. The first image is also used in the diagnosis and measurement of squint.

Much information regarding the changes in lens form during accommodation has also been obtained from the study of images III and IV.

10   Optics of Ametropia

In contrast to emmetropia (Chapter 9, pp. 107, 108) the ametropic eye fails to bring parallel light to a focus on the retina, i.e. the second principal focus of the eye does not fall on the retina.

Myopia

In the myopic eye, the second principal focus lies in front of the retina (Fig. 10.1). This may be because the eye is abnormally long. This is called *axial myopia* and includes high myopia in which there may be a posterior staphyloma.

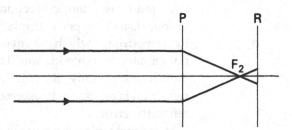

Fig. 10.1 Myopia.

Alternatively, the eye may be of normal length, but the dioptric power may be increased. This is called *refractive or index myopia*. Examples of this are keratoconus, where the corneal refractive power is increased, and nucleosclerosis, where the refractive power of the lens increases as the nucleus becomes more dense.

Hypermetropia

In the hypermetropic eye, the second principal focus lies behind the retina (Fig. 10.2).

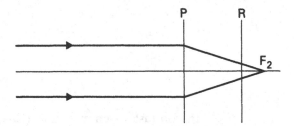

Fig. 10.2 Hypermetropia.

If the eye is short relative to its focal power, then *axial hypermetropia* results. Alternatively, if the refractive power of the eye is inadequate, then *refractive hypermetropia* results. Aphakia is an extreme example of refractive hypermetropia.

Phakic patients can overcome some or all of their hypermetropia by using accommodation for distance vision. They then have to exercise extra accommodation for near vision. Because the amplitude of accommodation declines with age (Chapter 11), these patients require reading glasses at a younger age than emmetropic patients.

Hypermetropia is classified into manifest and latent hypermetropia. *Manifest* hypermetropia is defined as the strongest convex lens correction accepted for clear distance vision. *Latent* hypermetropia is the remainder of the hypermetropia which is masked by ciliary tone and involuntary accommodation. This may account for several dioptres, especially in children, for whom cycloplegic refraction is necessary to ascertain the full magnitude of the refractive error.

Hypermetropia which can be overcome by accommodation is called *facultative*, while hypermetropia in excess of the amplitude of accommodation is called *absolute*.

Astigmatism

The refractive power of the astigmatic eye varies in different meridians. The image is formed as a Sturm's conoid (cf. Fig. 6.9).

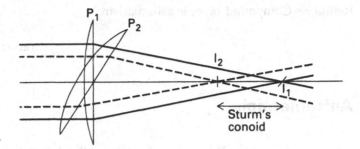

Fig. 10.3 Astigmatism; image formation.

If the principal meridians are at 90° to each other, this is called *regular astigmatism*. If the principal meridians are at 90° to each other but do not lie at or near 90° and 180°, the term *oblique astigmatism* is used. If the principal meridians are not at 90° to each other, this is called *irregular astigmatism* and cannot be corrected by spectacles.

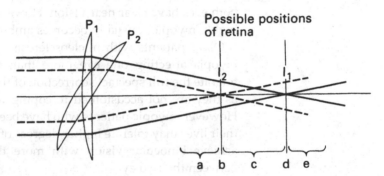

Fig. 10.4 Astigmatism; classification. Image position relative to retina.

Retina a = Compound hypermetropic astigmatism – rays in all meridians come to a focus behind the retina.

Retina b = Simple hypermetropic astigmatism – rays in one meridian focus on the retina, the other focus lies behind the retina.

Retina c = Mixed astigmatism – one line focus lies in front of the retina, the other behind the retina.

Retina d = Simple myopic astigmatism – one line focus lies on the retina, the other focus lies in front of the retina.

Retina e = Compound myopic astigmatism   – rays in all meridians come to a focus in front of the retina.

Anisometropia

When the refraction of the two eyes is different, the condition is known as *anisometropia*. Small degrees of anisometropia are commonplace. Larger degrees are a significant cause of amblyopia. A disparity of more than 1 D in the hypermetropic patient is enough to cause amblyopia of the more hypermetropic eye because accommodation is a binocular function, i.e. the individual eyes cannot accommodate by different amounts. The more hypermetropic eye therefore remains out of focus. The myopic patient with anisometropia is less likely to develop amblyopia because both eyes have clear near vision. However, when one eye is highly myopic it usually becomes amblyopic.

Older patients with nucleosclerosis and resulting index myopia affecting one eye more than the other may not tolerate the full spectacle correction of the more myopic eye as they are not accustomed to coping with anisometropia. However, myopic patients who have been anisometropic all their lives may tolerate higher degrees of anisometropia and achieve binocular vision with more than 2 D difference between the two eyes.

Pin-hole test

Because no focused image is formed on the retina of the ametropic eye, the visual acuity is reduced. The pin-hole test is a useful method of determining whether reduced visual acuity is due to refractive error rather than ocular pathology or neurological disease. If the visual acuity is reduced by refractive error, the pin-hole acuity will be significantly better than the unaided acuity. If the reduced acuity is due to ocular pathology, there is characteristically no improvement in visual acuity with the pin-hole. In macular disease the pin-hole acuity may be even worse than the unaided acuity.

The pin-hole theoretically allows only one ray from each point on an object to pass through to the screen. Thus, a clear image is formed regardless of the position of the screen (Fig. 10.5). Likewise the use of the ideal pin-hole leads to the formation of a clear retinal image irrespective of the refractive state of the eye.

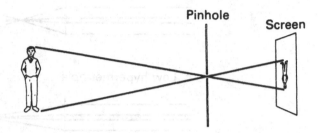

Fig. 10.5 Optical principle of the pin-hole.

But in practice the pin-holes available clinically allow a narrow pencil of light to pass through them, rather than a single ray.

Figure 10.6 shows that in low degrees of refractive error the pin-hole's effect is sufficient to improve the clarity of the retinal image to such an extent that a good visual acuity results. However, in high degrees of ametropia, although the pin-hole helps, the retinal image is still too diffuse to achieve the improvement that is found in the case of low refractive errors. Thus errors outside the range +4 D to –4 D sphere are not corrected to 6/6 with a pin-hole.

Stenopaeic slit

The stenopaeic slit can be used to determine the refraction and principal axes in astigmatism. The slit aperture acts as an elongated 'pin-hole', only allowing light in the axis of the slit to enter the eye. Hence, when the slit lies in one principal axis of the astigmatic eye, the second line focus is eliminated and the blur of Sturm's conoid reduced thus allowing a clearer image to be formed.

During the refraction of a patient with astigmatism, the slit is first rotated to a position in which the clearest vision is obtained. Spherical lenses are added to give further

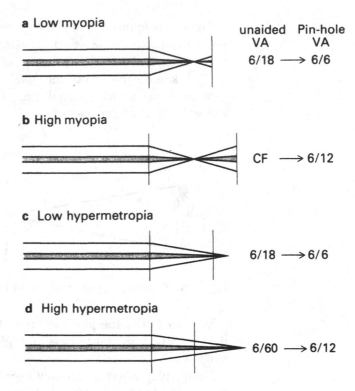

Fig. 10.6   Pin-hole: practical effect in ametropia.

improvement in acuity. The slit is then rotated through 90° and the spherical lens power adjusted to give best subjective acuity. The cylindrical correction required by the eye equals the algebraic difference between the two spherical corrections used, and its axis is that of the original direction of the slit.

In cases of corneal scarring, the stenopaeic slit may be used to determine the meridian along which the cornea is least deformed. In those cases where an optical iridectomy is indicated, this should be performed in this meridian.

Far point

The far point (FP) of an eye (Figs 10.7, 10.8 and 10.9) is the position of an object such that its image falls on the retina of the relaxed eye, i.e. in the absence of accommodation.

The distance of the far point from the principal plane of

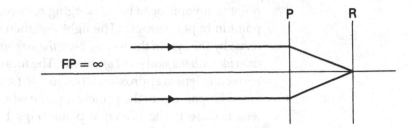

Fig. 10.7   The far point in emmetropia is infinity.

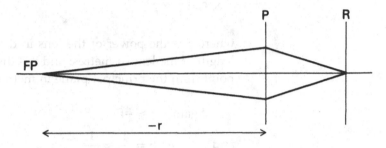

Fig. 10.8   The far point in myopia lies a finite distance in front of the eye.

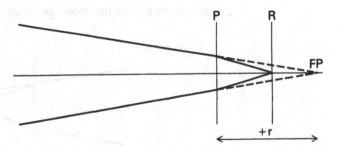

Fig. 10.9   The far point in hypermetropia is virtual, as only converging light can be focused on the retina.

the eye is denoted by r, which according to sign convention carries a negative sign in front of the principal plane and a positive sign behind the principal plane.

Optical correction of ametropia

The purpose of the correcting lens in ametropia is to deviate parallel incident light so that it appears to come from the far point in myopia or to be converging towards the virtual far point in hypermetropia. The light will then be brought to a focus by the eye on the retina. *Thus the far point of the eye must coincide with the focal point of the lens.* The focal length, f, of the correcting lens is approximately equal to ($\approx$) the distance, r, of the far point from the principal plane when the correcting lens is close to the principal plane (Figs 10.10 and 10.11). Thus the power of lens, F, required is

$$F = \frac{1}{f} \approx \frac{1}{r}$$

where F is the power of the lens in dioptres; f is the focal length of the lens in metres; and r is the distance of the far point from the principal plane in metres.

Again $- r \approx -f$

and $\qquad - F = \dfrac{1}{-f} \approx \dfrac{1}{-r}$

The reciprocal of the far point distance r, in metres, is symbolised by R, expressed in dioptres. R is known as the *static refraction* or the *ametropic error*.

a Uncorrected

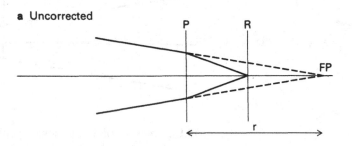

b Corrected

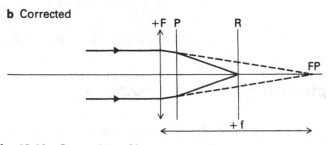

Fig. 10.10   Correction of hypermetropia.

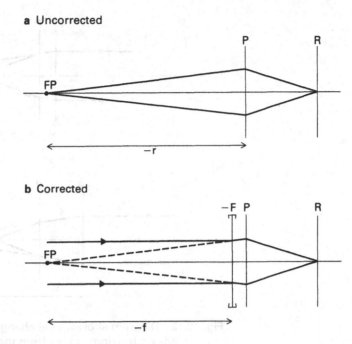

a Uncorrected

b Corrected

Fig. 10.11 Correction of myopia.

In practice, the correcting lens in ametropia is usually held in spectacles. The lens is, therefore, some distance in front of the principal plane of the eye. The power of the lens necessary to correct a specific degree of ametropia must therefore be adjusted so that the far point and the focus of the lens still coincide (see below, Effective power of lenses).

Effective power of lenses

If a correcting lens is moved either towards or away from the eye, its vergence power at the principal plane of the eye changes. The focus of the lens and the far point of the eye no longer coincide (Figs 10.12 and 10.13).

It can also be seen from the diagrams that, on moving either a convex or a concave lens away from the eye, the image is moved forward.

In the uncorrected hypermetropic eye (Fig. 10.2) the image falls behind the retina. The purpose of the correcting convex lens is to bring the image forward on to the retina. When the correcting lens is moved further away from the eye the image is brought still further forward. Thus the

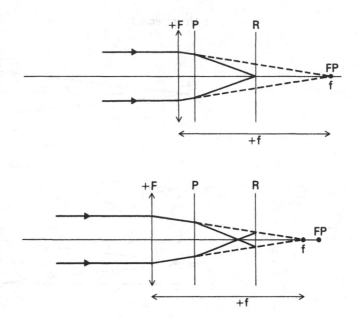

Fig. 10.12   Diagram showing the change in effectivity of a convex lens on moving it away from the eye.

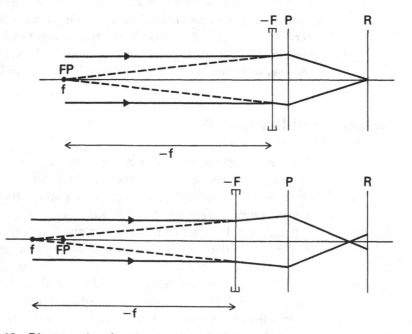

Fig. 10.13   Diagram showing the change in effectivity of a concave lens on moving it away from the eye.

effectivity of the lens is said to be increased. Therefore in this position a weaker convex lens throws the image onto the retina and corrects the hypermetropia.

In the myopic eye (Fig. 10.1) the image falls in front of the retina. The purpose of the correcting concave lens is to take the image back on to the retina. When the correcting lens is moved further away from the eye, the image moves forward again. Thus the effectivity of the lens is said to be reduced. Therefore, in this position, a stronger concave lens is needed to throw the image on to the retina.

In practice, patients with strong convex lenses, especially those who are aphakic, sometimes pull their glasses down their nose in order to read. The enhanced effectivity thus produced is sufficient to provide the reading correction. Also, myopes dislike their glasses slipping down their nose (as they tend to do if heavy glass lenses are used) as this makes the correction less effective.

Thus, to correct a specific degree of ametropia, the power of the correcting lens must be adjusted to take into account its position in front of the eye. A general formula exists for this purpose and applies to both convex and concave lenses.

Suppose a lens of focal length f_1 at a given position in front of the ametropic eye corrects the refractive error; then a different lens of focal length $(f_1 - d)$ is required when the correction is moved a distance d towards or away from the eye (Figs 10.14 and 10.15). The value of d is positive if the lens is moved towards the eye, and negative if moved away from the eye. The usual sign convention applies to the lens.

$$\text{Thus } F_2 = \frac{1}{f_1 - d}$$

where F_2 is the power of lens in dioptres required at the new position; f_1 is the focal length in metres of the original lens; and d is the distance moved in metres.

Mathematically the above formula can also be expressed as

$$F_2 = \frac{F_1}{1 - dF_1}$$

where F_1 is the dioptric power of the original lens.

a Spectacles

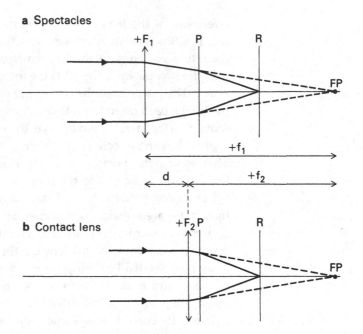

b Contact lens

Fig. 10.14 Correction of hypermetropia.

a Spectacles

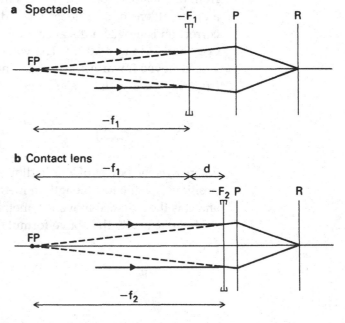

b Contact lens

Fig. 10.15 Correction of myopia.

Practical application: back vertex distance

For any lens of power greater than 5 dioptres, the position in front of the eye materially affects the optical correction of ametropia. This is especially true in aphakia where high power lenses are prescribed. For this reason the refractionist must state how far in front of the eye the trial lens is situated so that the dispensing optician can adjust the lens power if a contact lens is to be used, or if spectacles are to be worn at a different distance, e.g. because of a high-bridged nose or deep-set eyes.

Therefore any high powered lens should be placed in the back cell of the trial frame and the distance between the back of the lens and the cornea measured. This is called the *back vertex distance* (BVD) and must be given with all prescriptions over 5 dioptres. The measurement may be made with a ruler held parallel to the arm of the trial frame. Other means include a small rule which is slipped through a stenopaeic slit placed in the back cell of the trial frame until it touches the closed eyelid. Two millimetres must be added to the measurement to correct for the thickness of the lid.

Example 1 Refraction shows that an aphakic patient requires a +10.0 D lens at BVD 15 mm. He needs a contact lens (F_2)

$$F_2 = \frac{F_1}{1 - dF_1}$$

$$\text{Required power of contact lens} = F_2 = \frac{+10}{1 - 0.015 \times 10}$$

$$= \frac{+10}{1 - 0.15}$$

$$= \frac{+10}{0.85}$$

$$= +11.75 \text{ D}$$

Example 2 Likewise a high myope whose spectacle correction is –10.0 D at BVD 14 mm requires a contact lens (F_2)

$$F_2 = \frac{F_1}{1 - dF_1}$$

$$\text{Power of contact lens} = F_2 = \frac{-10}{1 - (+0.014 \times [-10])}$$

$$= \frac{-10}{1 - (0.14)}$$

$$= \frac{-10}{1.14}$$

$$= -8.75 \text{ D}$$

Happily, tables exist which give the value of F_2 when F_1 and d are known.

Spectacle magnification

The optical correction of ametropia is associated with a change in the retinal image size. The ratio between the corrected and uncorrected image size is known as the *spectacle magnification*.

$$\text{Spectacle magnification} = \frac{\text{corrected image size}}{\text{uncorrected image size}}$$

Clinically, it is more useful to compare the corrected ametropic image size with the emmetropic image size. This ratio is known as the *relative spectacle magnification* (RSM).

$$\text{Relative spectacle magnification} = \frac{\text{corrected ametropic image size}}{\text{emmetropic image size}}$$

In axial ametropia, if the correcting lens is placed at the anterior focal point of the eye, the image size is the same as in emmetropia. The RSM is therefore unity. However, in axial myopia (Fig. 10.16), if the correcting lens is worn nearer to the eye than the anterior focal point, the image size is increased. The relative spectacle magnification is therefore greater than unity. Contact lenses in axial myopia thus have a magnifying effect (Fig. 10.17).

In contrast to axial ametropia, the image size in refractive ametropia differs from the emmetropic image size even when the correcting lens is at the anterior focal point of the eye. The image size in refractive hypermetropia is increased, thus the relative spectacle magnification is greater than

Axial hypermetropia RSM = 1

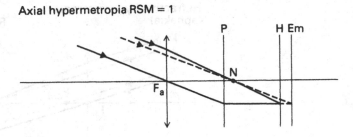

Axial myopia RSM = 1

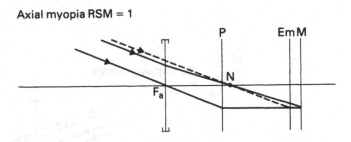

Fig. 10.16 Relative spectacle magnification. Axial ametropia with correcting lens at anterior focal point of the eye. Ametropic state (solid lines) compared with emmetropia (dotted lines).

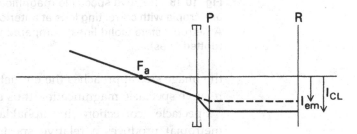

Fig. 10.17 Relative spectacle magnification. Axial myopia with correcting lens nearer the eye than the anterior focal point (contact lens). Ametropic state (solid lines) compared with emmetropia (dotted lines). I_{em} is the image size when correction is at the anterior focal point, which equals the emmetropic image size; and I_{CL} is the image size when correction is closer to the eye than the anterior focal point.

unity. In refractive myopia the image size is diminished, and thus the relative spectacle magnification is less than unity (Fig. 10.18).

Furthermore, in refractive ametropia, if the correcting lens is worn nearer to the eye than the anterior focal point,

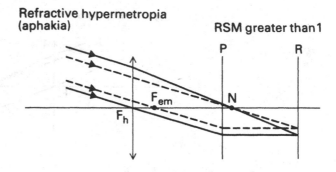

Refractive hypermetropia
(aphakia)   RSM greater than 1

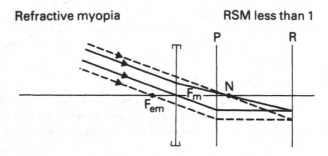

Refractive myopia   RSM less than 1

Fig. 10.18 Relative spectacle magnification. Refractive ametropia with correcting lens at anterior focal point of the eye. Ametropic state (solid lines) compared with emmetropia (dotted lines).

the image size approaches the emmetropic image size. The relative spectacle magnification thus approaches unity.

Spectacle correction in aphakia (refractive hypermetropia) produces a relative spectacle magnification of 1.36 when placed at the anterior focal point of the aphakic eye (23.2 mm in front of the principal plane) (see p. 105). However, when a contact lens is used, the relative spectacle magnification is reduced to 1.1 (Fig. 10.19). Spectacles are usually worn 12–15 mm in front of the cornea and the aphakic relative spectacle magnification at this position is approximately 1.33.

Calculation of RSM in aphakia when correcting lens is at the anterior focal point of the aphakic eye (Fig. 10.20)

Emmetropic anterior focal length, $F_{em}D = 17.05$ mm
Aphakic anterior focal length $F_{aph}D = 23.23$ mm

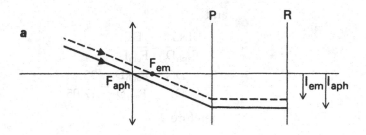

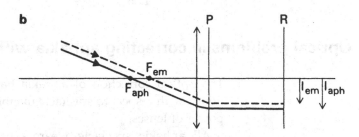

Fig. 10.19 Relative spectacle magnification: correction of aphakia with (a) spectacles at the anterior focal point, (b) contact lens. Ametropic state (solid lines) compared with emmetropia (dotted lines).

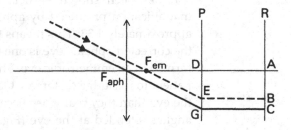

Fig. 10.20 Correction of aphakia with spectacles at anterior focal point. Ametropic state (solid lines) compared with emmetropia (dotted lines).

$$AB = DE = \text{emmetropic image size}$$
$$AC = DG = \text{corrected aphakic image size}$$

$$RSM = \frac{AC}{AB} = \frac{DG}{DE}$$

Since rays $F_{em}E$, and $F_{aph}G$ are parallel,

$$\text{angle } DF_{aph}G = \text{angle } DF_{em}E$$

and

$$\frac{DG}{F_{aph}D} = \frac{DE}{F_{em}D}$$

$$\frac{DG}{DE} = \frac{F_{aph}D}{F_{em}D} = \frac{23.23}{17.05}$$

Therefore

$$RSM = \frac{23.23}{17.05}$$

$$= 1.36$$

Optical problems in correcting aphakia with spectacles

The optical correction of aphakia has already been mentioned with respect to spectacle magnification and effective power of lenses.

All aphakic spectacle wearers have to contend with several problems due to the high refractive power of the lenses required (approx. + 10.0 D or more). The special problem of correcting unilateral aphakia in the presence of a normal fellow eye is discussed later.

It has been shown earlier that the relative spectacle magnification produced by aphakic spectacle correction is approximately 1.33. This means that the image produced in the corrected aphakic eye is one third larger than the image formed in an emmetropic eye. This magnification causes the patient to misjudge distances. Objects appear to be closer to the eye than they really are because of the increased visual angle subtended at the eye (Fig. 10.21). The image magnification also results in an enhanced performance of standard tests of visual acuity, e.g. Snellen test type. For example, a level of 6/9 for an aphakic spectacle wearer is equivalent to 6/12 for an emmetropic eye.

The use of a contact lens, or an intra-ocular implant, which reduces the RSM to 1.1 or 1.0 respectively, overcomes these problems.

The lenses used in aphakic spectacles are subject to the aberrations discussed in Chapter 8. In particular, image distortion is very troublesome to the newly aphakic patient. Straight lines appear curved except when viewed through a very small axial zone of the lens (pin cushion effect, p. 98). The linear environment thus appears as disconcerting

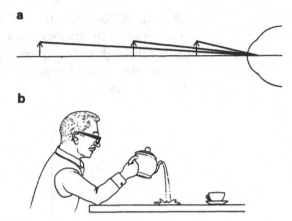

Fig. 10.21 (a) A standard object subtends a larger visual angle the closer it is to the eye. (b) An artificially magnified object is therefore assumed to be closer to the eye than it really is.

curves, and these change their shape as the patient moves his eyes and looks through different zones of his lenses. Patients usually adapt to this by learning to restrict their gaze to the axial zone of their lenses and by moving their head rather than their eyes to look around.

The prismatic effect (Chapter 5, p. 64) of aphakic spectacle lenses produces a ring scotoma all around the edge of the lens (Fig. 10.22). This scotoma may well cause patients to trip over unseen obstructions in their path.

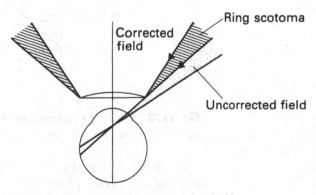

Fig. 10.22 Ring scotoma in corrected aphakia.

Furthermore, the direction of the ring scotoma changes as the patient moves his eyes, and objects may appear out of the scotoma or disappear into it – the 'jack-in-the-box' phenomenon.

Figure 10.23a shows the eye in the primary position and the location of the ring scotoma. An object O is visible to the patient through the periphery of the spectacle lens. Let us now consider what happens when the patient tries to look directly at object O.

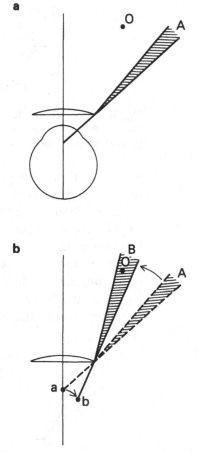

Fig. 10.23 Effect of eye movement on ring scotoma in corrected aphakia – jack-in-the-box phenomenon.

Reference to Fig. 10.23b shows that as the eye rotates, moving the nodal point from a to b, the ring scotoma moves in the opposite direction, from A to B. Thus when the patient tries to look at object O it disappears in the ring scotoma B only to reappear in his peripheral vision when he looks away. This disappearance and re-emergence of an object is known as the 'jack-in-the-box' phenomenon.

Finally, high powered glass lenses are heavy and may consequently cause the spectacles to slip down the patient's nose thus altering the effective power of the lenses. (Heavy spectacles are also uncomfortable to wear.) Weight may be reduced by the use of plastic lenses, but these tend to scratch especially if laid 'face' downwards when not in use. Another means of reducing lens weight and thickness is by the use of lenticular form lenses. A lenticular lens has only a central portion or aperture worked to prescription, the surrounding margin of the lens acting only as a carrier. However, the field of vision is necessarily reduced.

The foregoing aberrations and the prismatic effect and its consequences can all be eliminated by the use of contact lenses or intra-ocular implants. The advantages of these two forms of correction stem from the fact that in each case the correcting lens becomes an integral part of the optical system of the eye.

Correction of unilateral aphakia in the presence of a normal fellow eye

Spectacle correction of a unilateral aphakic eye can achieve a clear retinal image, but with an RSM of 1.33 the image in the aphakic eye is one third larger than the image in the normal fellow eye (Fig. 10.24). The patient is unable to fuse images of such unequal size (*aniseikonia*) and complains of seeing double.

The use of a contact lens or intra-ocular implant reduces the RSM to 1.1 or 1.0 respectively. The image in the aphakic eye will thus be the same size (intra-ocular implant) or only

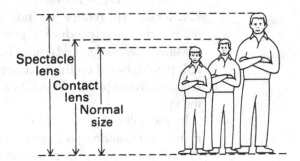

Spectacle lens

Contact lens

Normal size

Fig. 10.24 Relative spectacle magnification in corrected aphakia.

one tenth larger (contact lens). In either event the images can be fused and binocularity restored.

It is possible to produce a spectacle lens which has no focusing power but which alters retinal image size by increasing the visual angle subtended by an object at the eye (angular magnification, Chapter 5). Such a lens is called an *iseikonic lens*. The magnification depends on the curvature of the front surface of the lens and on its thickness. Thus, to produce pure magnification, the front curvature and lens thickness are calculated and the back curvature adjusted to render the lens afocal. Alternatively, a refractive correction may be imposed on such a lens. However, the maximum magnification which can be achieved in practice by an iseikonic lens is only about 5%, which is insufficient to be of practical benefit in the correction of unilateral aphakia.

Iseikonic lenses have been used to treat other causes of aniseikonia (different retinal image size in the two eyes), but they have fallen into disuse for several reasons. They are expensive, requiring to be individually made on special machinery. Also, they are thick and heavy to wear.

Correction of aphakia with an intra-ocular lens

The insertion of an intra-ocular lens (IOL) within the aphakic eye overcomes the optical disadvantages of aphakic spectacles and the handling and wearing difficulties encountered with contact lenses. The IOL becomes part of the optical system of the eye, and because it is situated at or very close to the position of the crystalline lens, problems with RSM do not arise.

Preoperatively, it is desirable to predict the power of the IOL which will render the individual patient emmetropic or, in some cases, produce a desired refractive error.

Many *theoretical formulae* have been devised for predicting IOL power, based on the calculation of the vergence power required in the plane of the IOL at a known position within the eye.

In the following reasoning a = axial length of globe in metres; k = pseudophakic anterior chamber depth in metres; P_c = refractive power of cornea in dioptres; and n = index of refraction of aqueous and vitreous.

At the IOL, light must have a vergence equal to the

dioptric value of the distance (a–k) between the IOL and the retina if the focus is to fall on the retina. Because the IOL is not in air, the distance (a–k) must be divided by n, the refractive index of the aqueous and vitreous. The dioptric value of this therefore equals n/(a – k). The vergence power in the plane of the IOL will be the combined effect of the refractive power of the IOL and the cornea. The effective power of the cornea in the plane of the IOL is calculated using the effective power of lenses formula, $F_2 = F_1/(1 - dF_1)$. Substituting P_c for F_1, and k/n for d (because the distance k is in aqueous of refractive index n), the effective power of the cornea in the plane of the IOL will be

$$\frac{P_c}{1 - \dfrac{P_c.k}{n}}$$

Therefore

Required = required vergence – effective power of
IOL power   in plane of IOL   cornea in plane of IOL

$$= \frac{n}{a-k} - \frac{P_c}{1 - \dfrac{P_c.k}{n}}$$

A more pragmatic approach to the problem of predicting IOL power is to look at the refractive results obtained in clinical practice and work back from them to a formula.

Analysis of data obtained from such retrospective study of large numbers of eyes in which IOLs have been implanted has resulted in the *regression analysis intraocular lens formula*. In 1980 Sanders, Retzlaff and Kraff further simplified this formula, producing what has become known as the *SRK formula*.

The SRK formula states that

$$P = A - B(AL) - C(K)$$

where P is the IOL power in dioptres; A is a constant which reflects the position of the particular model of IOL within the eye; B is the multiplication constant for the axial length; AL is the axial length in mm; C is the multiplication constant for the average keratometry reading; K is the average keratometry reading in dioptres; and the values of the multiplication constants are B = 2.5 and C = 0.9.

Substituting

$$P = A - (2.5 \times \text{axial length}) - (0.9 \times \text{average keratometry})$$
$$\qquad\qquad \text{in mm} \qquad\qquad\qquad \text{in dioptres}$$

If a refractive condition (R) other than emmetropia is desired, the formula is modified to become

$$P = A - B(AL) - C(K) - D(R)$$

where D is the multiplication constant for the desired refraction. The value for D is 1.25 if the IOL power for emmetropia is greater than 14 D, and 1.0 if the IOL power for emmetropia is less than or equal to 14 D.

If the IOL power has been calculated for a posterior chamber lens and at surgery an anterior chamber lens has to be used, the required IOL power must be reduced by the difference in the A constants of the IOLs. This is because the anterior chamber lens lies further forward in the eye and therefore has a lower A constant. The equivalent anterior chamber IOL is usually 2 dioptres weaker than the posterior chamber lens.

The original SRK formula was found to be inaccurate for eyes of short (less than 22 mm) or long (24.5 mm or above) axial length. The SRK II formula, introduced in 1988, incorporates the following correction. The A constant is adjusted (and termed A1) in a step-wise way over the range of axial lengths.

For axial lengths of

less than 20 mm,	A1 = A + 3
20 mm to less than 21 mm,	A1 = A + 2
21 mm to less than 22 mm,	A1 = A + 1
22 mm to less than 24.5 mm,	A1 = A
24.5 mm and above,	A1 = A − 0.5

The SRK II formula is easy to use and is widely employed in clinical practice. A further refinement, the theoretical SRK (SRK-T) formula, has been devised to improve the accuracy when very high or very low IOL powers are required.

In order to apply any SRK formula, the keratometry and axial length of the individual eye must be known. The corneal curvature and hence its refractive power is measured using a keratometer (Chapter 14) while the axial length is measured by A-scan ultrasonography.

Sound and ultrasound energy are transmitted by the vibration of adjacent particles and travel faster the more dense the medium. Like light, the energy is reflected at interfaces between media of different acoustic density. A probe emitting pulses of ultrasound is lightly applied to the cornea. The ultrasound passes through the eye and is reflected from the posterior corneal surface, the anterior and posterior surfaces of the lens and the retina and sclera. The pulse-echo times are recorded and, since the speeds of ultrasound in the various ocular media are known, the axial length may be calculated. A correction factor must be applied if the vitreous has been replaced by silicone oil.

A-scan ultrasound may also be used to measure corneal thickness.

To accurately predict IOL power, it is essential to measure the axial length along the visual axis of the eye. Measurements at other orientations will be shorter and as the axial length is multiplied by a factor of 2.5 in the SRK formula it is the major source of error in the clinical calculation of IOL power. Both eyes should be measured as this helps to expose any error. Error should be suspected and the measurements checked in the following circumstances: if the axial lengths are very different (more than 0.5 mm difference) in the absence of clinical anisometropia, or seem inappropriate to the refractive state of the eye, or if the predicted post-operative refraction is not achieved in the first eye. The highly myopic eye with a posterior staphyloma poses a particular problem as it is all too easy to measure the axial length to the edge of the staphyloma, especially as the full depth of the staphyloma may be beyond the range of measurement of some A-scan machines. In this situation a B-scan (a two-dimensional ultrasound scan) will allow imaging of the shape of the eye, including the staphyloma, and the axial length can be measured from the image.

A wise choice of desired post-operative refraction for the individual patient is crucial in the calculation of IOL power.

Not all patients will be happy to be rendered emmetropic or –1.00 D myopic. In general, the following factors should be taken into consideration.

- The state of the fellow eye. If this has good acuity, either having no significant cataract, or being pseudophakic, it is important to avoid significant anisometropia and all the problems that go with it, namely aniseikonia and disruption of binocular vision (cf. p. 19).
- The patient's previous refractive experience. On the whole, life-long myopes do not like having to use convex reading glasses, and prefer to use a concave distance correction.

Multifocal IOLs are available, but are not yet in general use. The simplest work by providing two lens powers, for distance and near vision. More complex designs offer intermediate powers increasing the depth of focus.

Unlike multifocal spectacles which have differing power at different zones of the lens (Chapter 11) so that only one zone and power are used at a time, multifocal IOLs form multiple images over the whole lens aperture. In the case of bifocal IOLs, two images of an object are formed, one of which will fall on the retina when the object is at infinity, the other falling on the retina when the object is at the patient's reading distance. Neither image is as clear and bright as that formed by a monofocal IOL. Furthermore, the second image forms a blur-circle on the retina which may degrade the perceived clarity of vision and cause glare when bright objects are viewed, e.g. when driving at night. This effect differs with different lens designs.

The following optical principles are employed in IOL design to achieve a multifocal effect. Concentric zones of graded power are used in some designs, the near zone being at or close to the centre because the pupil constricts for near vision. This may cause difficulty for distance vision in bright light. To overcome this problem another design relies on concentric annular zones, each of which has graded near to distance power, to provide near and distance correction over the whole lens aperture. Alternatively, diffraction of light (see Chapter 1) from multiple ring steps worked on the posterior surface of a distance power IOL may be used to provide the second image for near vision by constructive interference between waves of light diffracted by the various zones of the lens.

Refractive state after removal of the crystalline lens from a highly myopic eye

The patient with a highly myopic eye who undergoes cataract extraction represents a special case. The removal of the converging power of the crystalline lens reduces the total refractive power of the eye. If the degree of axial myopia is equal and opposite to the effective power of the removed lens, the eye is rendered emmetropic and the patient can see distant objects clearly without spectacles (see Fig. 10.25). This occurs after cataract extraction in axial myopia of –18 D to –20 D.

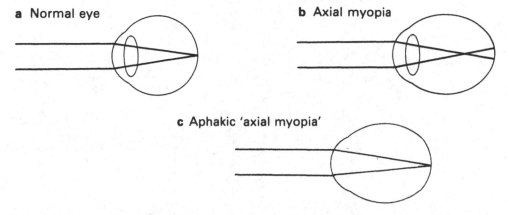

Fig. 10.25   Refractive effect of aphakia in axial myopia of –18 D to –20 D.

It should be recalled that the effective power of the crystalline lens *in situ* is only +15 D. It might be supposed therefore that axial myopia of –15 D would be corrected by removing the crystalline lens. But because of the change in effectivity of lenses, in order to achieve a correction of –15 D in the plane of the crystalline lens, a spectacle correction of –15 D to –20 D is required. (The exact requirement depends upon the individual characteristic of the eye in question – cf. variable states of emmetropia, Chapter 9.) Because the degree of myopia is referred to by the strength of spectacle correction, it is the myope of –18 D to –20 D who becomes emmetropic after cataract extraction.

It will be recalled that the actual power of the crystalline lens in isolation is +19 D although it only contributes +15 D to the overall refractive power of the eye. Standard intra-ocular implant lenses are therefore usually of approxi-mately +19 D power.

11   Presbyopia

Definition of presbyopia

The amplitude of accommodation declines steadily with age. This is due mainly to sclerosis of the fibres of the crystalline lens and changes in its capsule which reduce the spontaneous steepening of its surfaces when the ciliary muscle contracts. Also it may be that the ciliary muscle itself becomes less efficient with advancing age (after 40 years).

In infancy the eye is capable of 14 D of accommodation, but by the age of 45 years this has fallen to about 4 D. After the age of 60 years only 1 D or less remains, and part of this is probably due to depth of field, which may be enhanced by senile miosis. (A patient with no accommodation will have 0.25 D depth of field, enabling him to see clearly from 4 metres to infinity.)

In order to focus on an object at a reading distance of 25 cm, the emmetropic eye must accommodate by 4 D (see Chapter 9). However, for comfortable near vision one-third of the available accommodation must be kept in reserve. Therefore, the patient will begin to experience difficulty or discomfort for near vision at 25 cm when his accommodation has decayed to 6 D. This usually occurs between 40 and 45 years of age. A person experiencing such difficulty and discomfort for near vision due to reduced amplitude of accommodation is said to be *presbyopic*. A supplementary convex lens is used to enable the patient to achieve comfortable near vision. The lens is called a *presbyopic correction* and the age-related inadequacy of accommodation is called *presbyopia*.

Presbyopia cannot be defined in terms of remaining amplitude of accommodation because the onset of symptoms varies with the patient's preferred working distance, the nature of the close work and the length of time for which it is done.

Calculation of presbyopic correction

The amount of presbyopic correction necessary for a given patient can be calculated if the remaining amplitude of accommodation is determined (from his near point) and the desired working distance is specified. For example, an emmetropic patient has a remaining amplitude of accommodation of 3 D (near point 33 cm). In order to achieve comfortable near vision he must keep one third of this in reserve. Therefore, he must use only 2 D of his 3 D of accommodation. If he wishes to see clearly at 25 cm he needs 4 D of accommodation. Thus he requires a presbyopic correction of 2 D.

In practice the refractionist learns by experience to anticipate the approximate presbyopic correction from the patient's age (see Chapter 16, p. 237). This is then confirmed by subjective refraction. In ametropia the presbyopic correction is added to the patient's distance correction.

The onset of presbyopia occurs earlier in uncorrected hypermetropia than in emmetropia, because the patient with hypermetropia must accommodate more to achieve near vision. For example, a patient with 3 D of hypermetropia needs to exert 3 D of accommodation to see clearly at infinity. Therefore, to see clearly at 25 cm 7 D of accommodation are needed (3 D + 4 D) (Fig. 11.1). Con-

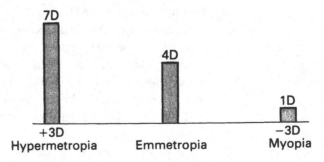

Fig. 11.1 Amplitude of accommodation necessary to achieve clear vision at 25 cm in different refractive states.

versely a patient with 3D of myopia has a far point at 33 cm. Thus to focus at 25 cm only 1D of accommodation is used.

Figure 11.2 relates the three refractive states shown in Fig. 11.1 to the decline of amplitude of accommodation with age. It is apparent that the onset of presbyopia occurs earlier in uncorrected hypermetropia than in emmetropia and in uncorrected myopia it is delayed. Furthermore, in myopia of 4D or more the patient can always read without glasses. However, many myopic patients prefer to use bifocal or multifocal spectacles for convenience, and to overcome any astigmatism or anisometropia that may be present.

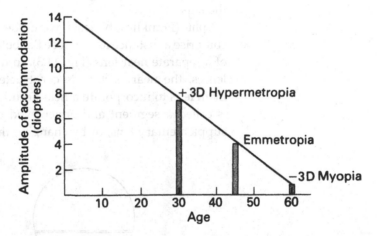

Fig. 11.2 Decline in amplitude of accommodation with increasing age.

The presbyopic correction must be adjusted for different working distances. A patient may require mid-distance glasses, e.g. for reading music, as well as for reading text.

In practice it is easy to prescribe too strong a presbyopic correction for a given task because the patient, away from his or her usual surroundings and anxious to perform well, tends to hold the reading test type closer to the eyes than usual. A useful safeguard against over-correction is to ensure that the patient can read N5 at his or her approximate reading distance but also N8 at arm's length with the proposed correction.

Multifocal lenses

It is often inconvenient for the presbyopic patient to have separate pairs of distance and reading spectacles, and there is considerable demand for single lenses which incorporate both the distance and near correction.

Bifocal lenses

A single pair of spectacles with bifocal lenses provides separate distance and near prescriptions for each eye. The distance portion is usually the larger of the two – the major portion. The near portion usually occupies the lower part of the lens.

Split (Franklin) bifocals were the earliest design and comprise a distance lens whose flat bottom abuts the flat top of a separate near lens (Fig. 11.3). In newer types of bifocal lenses, the near portion is constructed by modifying the main lens to incorporate a near addition. This modification is called a segment and is achieved either by attaching a supplementary lens, or by changing the surface curvature.

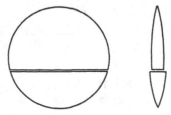

Fig. 11.3   Split bifocal lens – Franklin design.

Cemented bifocals have a near portion constructed by attaching a supplementary lens to the surface of a distance lens of the same refractive index (Fig. 11.4). Ultraviolet-cured epoxy resin has superseded Canada balsam (a tree resin) as the adhesive. The segment edge of a wafer bifocal is almost imperceptibly thin on the rear surface and the bifocal lens appears as if it were a single piece of glass. However, this lens design is now almost obsolete.

In fused bifocals, the near portion is made by heat-fusing a button of flint glass to a corresponding depression in a

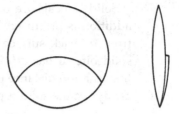

Fig. 11.4 Cemented wafer bifocal lens.

crown glass main lens which has a lower refractive index (Fig. 11.5). A flat top segment is made using a composite button, where the top of the button is made of crown glass and merges with the main lens once heat-fused. The button is then ground to make the surface curvature of the segment the same as that of the distance portion. Different types of flint glass allow variation in the refractive index and power of the segment. The near addition therefore depends on the refractive index of each glass type, and the surface curvatures of the depression and the distance portion. The higher refractive index of a fused bifocal segment may cause chromatic aberration near the segment edge. Cemented and fused segments can be made in different shapes to suit occupational requirements (Fig. 11.6).

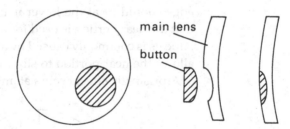

Fig. 11.5 Fused bifocal lens.

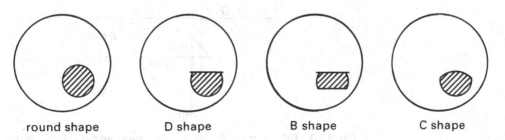

round shape   D shape   B shape   C shape

Fig. 11.6 Segment shapes for right eye fused bifocal lenses.

Solid bifocals are of single piece construction. The near addition is produced by a different curvature of either the front or back surface of this portion. The executive-style solid bifocal has a full-width horizontal junction between the near and distance portions (Fig. 11.7). Plastic bifocals are always of the solid type.

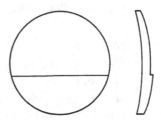

Fig. 11.7 Solid bifocal (executive).

The distance (DVP) and near (NVP) visual points are positions on a lens through which it is assumed the visual axis is directed while the spectacles are in use. The NVP is 2 mm nasal to and 8 mm below the DVP (Fig. 11.8). The top of the near portion should be tangential with the inferior limbus of the cornea for most purposes. When prescribing for children, for whom executive bifocals may be prescribed to overcome convergence excess esotropia, the segment edge should be at the lower margin of the pupil to ensure that the near portion is used for all near tasks. Intolerance of bifocals is commonly caused by a poorly fitting frame which allows the near portion to slip too low for comfortable use.

A prismatic effect occurs at any non-axial point on a lens

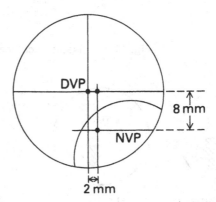

Fig. 11.8 Bifocal lens. Position of the near and distance visual points.

(see p. 64, spherical lens decentration). If the optical centre of each portion of the lens coincides with the NVP or DVP, it follows that an increasing prismatic effect occurs towards the junction of the distance and near portions. The prism power at the junction will suddenly change when the patient looks from one portion to the other and the image will suddenly change position – *prismatic jump*; (the prism power is proportional to the dioptric power of each portion and the distance of the interface from its optical centre). A second optical consideration with bifocal lenses is the prismatic effect at the NVP. This is the sum of the prismatic effect due to the main lens and that due to the segment at this point (Fig. 11.9). For most fused or cemented segment bifocals, the optical centre of the segment overlies the NVP of the main lens and produces no extra prismatic effect beyond that caused by looking through an eccentric point on the distance lens (Fig. 11.6). Bifocals may not be tolerated by patients with anisometropia because the prismatic effect on each eye will be different. More than 1.5 prism dioptres of vertical prismatic imbalance may be insuperable and make binocular vision uncomfortable or cause diplopia. High refractive errors magnify the imbalance and, in addition, the large prismatic effect they induce may require an uncomfortable degree of down-gaze in order to read. Prismatic jump and excessive prismatic effect at the NVP are therefore most troublesome in higher-powered lenses. Great care must also be exercised when prescribing for patients with vertical extraocular muscle imbalance.

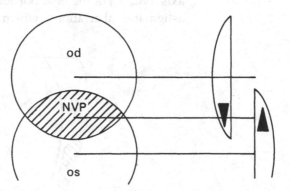

Fig. 11.9 The prismatic effect at the NVP is the sum of that due to the main lens and the downcurve segment at that point. od, os: Optical centres of distance portion and downcurve bifocal segment.

Prismatic jump can be reduced if the optical centres of the lens lie at or near the junction of the two portions. In a monocentric (executive) bifocal, they coincide at the junction of the distance and near portions and no prismatic jump occurs. Shaped segments reduce jump because the segment top is only a short distance from its optical centre. A down-curve circular segment has a base-down prismatic effect at the NVP because its optical centre is always below it (Fig. 11.9). This counters the base-up effect of a hypermetropic distance correction but adds to the base-down effect of a myopic distance correction which may make it intolerable. Alternatively, image jump and prismatic effect are reduced by incorporating a base-up prism in the near segment. Any bifocals designed to counter prismatic effect may be described as *prism controlled*, although the term is often used only where this is achieved by incorporation of a prism. Prismatic correction may be pre-cast, or, in straight-top fused or cemented bifocals a *biprism (slab-off)* process may be employed (Fig. 11.10). First, a prismatic correction is added to the near and distance portions of the less prismatic lens in order that the prismatic effect at the NVP of each is equal. Base-up prism is then removed from the upper part of the modified lens so that the original prismatic modification affects only the near portion. The biprism process is useful where anisometropia causes excessive vertical prismatic imbalance at the NVP.

Another optical problem with bifocal lenses is that the near visual axis (NR) does not correspond with the optical axis (NC^{1}C^3) of the near portion of the lens (Fig. 11.11). The astigmatic aberrations which occur when light passes

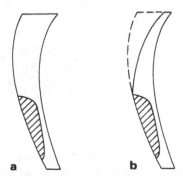

a   b

Fig. 11.10   The biprism process. Base-up prism is incorporated with the prescription (a). It is then removed from the distance portion only (b).

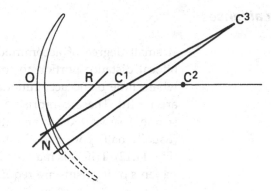

Fig. 11.11 Bifocal lens. This shows the visual axes and optical axes of the lens. O, Distance visual point; N, near visual point; R, centre of rotation of the eye; C^1, centre of front surface of lens; C^2, centre of back surface of lens; C^3, centre of near segment back surface.

obliquely through a lens are therefore present to some degree when the near portion is used (see p. 115, oblique astigmatism). To reduce this astigmatism, bifocal spectacles should be made so that the top of each lens is tilted forward 10 to 20° (pantoscopic tilt) making the visual axis more perpendicular to the near portion of the lens when reading (see Fig. 8.9a). Otherwise, in strong prescriptions, looking through the lens obliquely will induce additional cylindrical effects and aberrations.

When prescribing bifocals it is important to consider the needs of the individual patient. A typist or supermarket cashier needs to view a relatively large area at a slightly greater distance than the usual reading distance. The near portion should therefore be large and have a reduced presbyopic correction. On the other hand, a person working outdoors who does little near work benefits from a smaller near segment. Occupations involving work at a height, for example on scaffolding, are a contraindication for bifocals because down-gaze will be dangerous through the near portion. Because there is a distorted, blurred and prismatically displaced view of the ground through the near portion, bifocals are also unsuitable for elderly people unsteady on their feet or suffering from vertigo.

Emmetropic patients are often suited by half glasses comprising a presbyopic correction alone. Conversely, the low myope may choose a lens with the power portion cut away to enable him to read with the naked eye.

Trifocal lenses

A small degree of accommodation may allow use of the bifocal distance portion to focus for middle distance, but where little or no accommodation remains, trifocal lenses are useful. These comprise a distance portion and a near segment separated by an intermediate segment of lesser (usually half) power to allow clear middle distance vision (Fig. 11.12). Trifocals may not be tolerated by anisometropic patients or if prisms are required for near work.

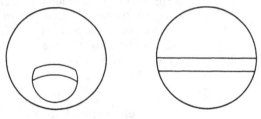

Fig. 11.12   Trifocal lenses.

Progressive addition lenses

The lens power of progressive addition lenses (PALs) changes gradually between the distance and near visual points so that a single pair of spectacles suffices for all distances. There is no visible interface between distance and near portions and this avoids the cosmetic disadvantages of a segment edge crossing the eye.

Between the DVP and NVP is the power progression corridor, where the lens is optically true and focuses for intermediate distances (Fig. 11.13). This avoids the sudden step in power or prism occurring at the interface as in conventional multifocal lenses. To each side of the progression corridor, aberration and astigmatism increase peripherally and may be intolerable for prescriptions with a large cylinder or high reading addition. Lens designs are often unique to a manufacturer. Some older designs only achieve the full reading addition near the lower edge of the lens. In dispensing such a lens it is wise to specify an extra +0.50 D added to the near addition prescription to ensure that sufficient reading power is present at the NVP.

PALs vary between 'hard' and (newer) 'soft' and 'ultra soft' designs. 'Hard' designs have relatively wide distance

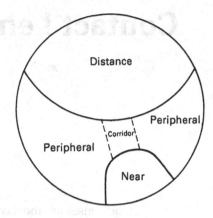

Fig. 11.13 Progressive power lens.

and near portions, but the progression corridor is narrow and aberrations occur close to it. Newer 'soft' designs have smaller distance and near portions, allowing a wider progression corridor with less pronounced aberrations to each side; they are therefore better tolerated. Patients requiring a wide near portion are unlikely to succeed with PALs.

12   Contact Lenses

Contact lenses are most commonly worn as an alternative to spectacles by those who perceive the wearing of spectacles to be unattractive or inconvenient. They are safer than spectacles for many sports and occupations because they do not fall off, break, fog up, become spattered in rain or impair the use of protective eye wear. Contact lenses are optically superior to spectacles in some cases. They reduce or eliminate the aberrations associated with spectacles used to correct high refractive errors. They also reduce the aniseikonia associated with anisometropia and high degrees of astigmatism.

Contact lenses are used diagnostically and during surgery to view the fundus and trabecular meshwork. A number of non-refracting contact lenses are used in ophthalmology: bandage contact lenses (precorneal membranes) are used therapeutically for ocular surface disorders to protect and promote healing and to relieve pain. A painted contact lens may be worn to improve the appearance of a small or an unsightly blind eye and to provide an artificial iris in aniridia. A type of contact lens with an attached electrode is used to perform electroretinography (ERG).

Geometry

The refracting power of the optical (central) zone of a contact lens is determined by its anterior and posterior curvatures, thickness and refractive index. A contact lens is described as spherical when it has the same radius of surface curvature in each meridian. Cylindrical refractive errors may be corrected by contact lenses in which the front surface, back surface or both are toric (cf. Chapter 6, pp. 70, 71). Torsion of a toric contact lens may be prevented either by incorporating an up to 2.00 D base-down prism to weight the lower pole of the lens, or by removing the lower 0.5–1 mm of the lens (truncation) to allow it to sit on the edge of the lower eyelid.

The posterior surface of the optical zone is defined by its posterior central curvature (PCC), also known as the base curve. The base curve is measured by its radius in millimetres or by its dioptric power in air. The shape of the posterior surface curvature of a contact lens should conform closely to the aspheric surface of the cornea (cf. p. 93) to ensure a correct fit. An aspheric shape may be created by encircling the optical zone with one or two concentric zones of increasing radius of curvature to produce a bicurve or tricurve contact lens; the junctions between the zones are made smooth by a process called blending. This has been superseded by computer-controlled production of a precise aspheric curve. The base curve and the diameter of the contact lens determine how tightly the lens fits the cornea and how easily it moves with each blink.

Corneal contact lenses have a smaller diameter than the cornea on which they are supported. Scleral (haptic) contact lenses have a peripheral rim which is supported by the sclera; they are now rarely used, although they are easier to handle because of their large (25 mm) diameter. The corneal surface is oxygenated by the tear film. Contact lenses made of gas-impermeable materials may therefore incorporate fenestrations, slots or grooves to facilitate the circulation of tears behind the lens.

Contact lenses used to correct high refractive errors present problems because of their greater thickness and weight. The tendency of the upper eyelid to grip the thick upper edge of a high power minus (concave) lens and cause it to ride high is countered by a peripheral bevel. The weight of a high power (convex) plus lens that causes it to drop to a lower position can be countered by a minus peripheral carrier portion which tends to be lifted by the upper lid.

Tear lens and astigmatism

The refractive index of the precorneal tear film (1.333) almost equals that of the cornea (1.3375). Optically, the tear film neutralises corneal surface irregularity, and the refractive power of the corneal surface is effectively that of the tear film–air interface.

The tear film between the posterior surface of a contact lens and the anterior surface of the cornea is known as the tear lens. If it has uniform thickness it has plano power. A steeper base curve (that is, a more vaulted contact lens) increases the axial height of the tear lens to make it more strongly positive; the converse makes it more negative. The tear lens allows a spherical contact lens to neutralise corneal astigmatism. The base curve of the contact lens should be the same as the corneal surface curvature in the flattest meridian, so that where the cornea is steeper the tear lens is thicker and neutralises the astigmatism. It is therefore convenient to express the prescription using negative cylindrical powers because only the spherical component need be prescribed.

Whereas rigid lenses can normally correct large degrees of corneal astigmatism, soft contact lenses neutralise no more than 1.00 D in this way because they tend to adopt the shape of the cornea. Corneal astigmatism of more than 1.50–2.00 D is therefore an important limitation to the use of soft contact lenses. Astigmatism arising from the crystalline lens or an implanted intraocular lens will only be neutralised by a front surface toric contact lens.

Differences between contact lenses and spectacles

Field of view

A contact lens moves with the eye and therefore allows good vision in all positions of gaze. The distortions which occur when looking through the periphery of a spectacle lens do not occur. When the pupil is dilated, a rigid contact lens may cause a halo effect because of refraction through the peripheral zone of the lens or adjacent tear film.

Hypermetropic patients reduce their field of view by wearing spectacles because the lens periphery has a prismatic effect with the base towards the visual axis. When they change to contact lenses they do not need to move their eyes so far to see the same overall field of view. The opposite applies to myopic patients whose spectacles increase the field of view because of a prismatic effect with the base away from the visual axis.

Aspects of image magnification associated with contact lens wear are described elsewhere (cf. spectacle magnification, p. 126). Most anisometropia is axial, and changing from spectacles to contact lenses in such cases produces image magnification (and improved visual acuity) for myopic patients and image minification for those who are hypermetropic. Aniseikonia is reduced with contact lenses compared with spectacles (cf. p. 133, Fig. 10.24).

Optical aberration

Correct contact lens fitting ensures that the lens remains almost centred in all positions of gaze and that on blinking any lens movement is not excessive. This minimises the oblique aberration which occurs looking through non-axial portions of the lens (cf. Aberrations of optical systems, p. 95) and allows good visual acuity in peripheral gaze.

Accommodation and convergence

Spectacle lenses which are centred for distance induce a prismatic effect when the eyes converge for near vision. No such effect occurs with contact lenses, which remain centred. Myopic spectacles have a base–in prismatic effect which reduces the amount of convergence and accommodation required for near (cf. AC:A ratio, p. 110). A change to contact lenses therefore demands greater convergence and accommodation which may cause eye strain in presbyopic myopes (cf. Fig. 12.1). The unequal prismatic effect of anisometropic spectacles is eliminated by contact lenses.

Prisms

It is possible to incorporate up to 3 dioptres of prism power into a corneal contact lens without making it too thick to be practical. The weight of the prism rotates the contact lens so that the prism is always base down. This makes horizontal

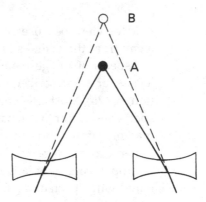

Fig. 12.1 Myopic spectacle base-in effect. The visual axis is directed towards B when looking at a near object A.

prismatic correction impossible and limits the prism to one lens only. Carefully fitted scleral lenses allow incorporation of vertical or horizontal prism up to 6 prism dioptres divided between the two lenses.

Tint

Contact lenses may incorporate a slight blue tint to make them more visible for easier handling and retrieval. They may also have a deeper green, blue or brown tint (sparing the centre) to make the iris appear a different colour.

Bifocal contact lenses

Presbyopic, pseudophakic and aphakic patients need to achieve optical correction for more than one object distance because their accommodation is reduced or absent (cf. Chapter 11). The contact lens alternatives available to these patients without accommodation are the wearing of spectacles over contact lenses, bifocal contact lenses or monovision. Monovision entails fitting one eye (usually the one with better vision) with a distance contact lens and the fellow eye with a lens which corrects the near vision. Patients must learn to adapt to having to concentrate on the clearer image from one eye. Binocularity and stereopsis are diminished.

Various bifocal and multifocal contact lens designs are available: annular, aspheric, segmental and diffractive. Annular bifocal contact lenses have a central zone which usually corrects for distance, surrounded by an annular zone for near. In down gaze, the contact lens rises relative to the cornea, placing the near portion in front of the visual axis.

Light from a distant object that passes through the portion of the lens which focuses for distance produces a clear retinal image. However, under these circumstances, the light passing through the near portion of the contact lens produces a superimposed out-of-focus image. The blurred image reduces the quality of the clear one. The reverse applies when viewing a near object. The wearer learns to concentrate on the better focused image. A major drawback of annular bifocals is that the peripheral (annular) portion of the lens is not as effective when the pupil diameter is small.

In an aspheric multifocal contact lens the central part of the lens corrects for distance and there is a gradual transition in power to the peripheral portion which corrects for near. Only a small amount of the total light entering the eye through the contact lens is in focus on the retina and this must compete with a blurred image from light passing through other parts of the contact lens as described above.

Segmental bifocal contact lenses incorporate the near addition over the lower portion of the lens. The eye looks through the distance portion in the primary position. In down gaze, the contact lens rises relative to the cornea, placing the near portion in front of the visual axis. Segmented bifocals must be prevented from rotating by truncation (Fig. 12.2) or by ballasting with a base-down prism.

Diffractive bifocal lenses have concentric diffraction rings on their posterior surface which are designed to focus equal amounts of light from distant and near objects. The image is

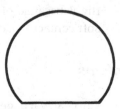

Fig. 12.2 Truncated contact lens.

less bright than with a single-focus contact lens and this may be a problem in dim illumination.

Keratoconus

The increased corneal surface curvature in keratoconus causes increasing myopia and irregular astigmatism. Mild cases are amenable to spectacle correction but myopia and astigmatism frequently progress to the extent that only rigid contact lenses allow satisfactory vision. Historically, haptic contact lenses were used but newer corneal lenses are designed to sit on the cone. In severe keratoconus when the cone is too steep or scarred, contact lenses may not be appropriate and corneal grafting may be necessary.

Other optical problems associated with contact lens wear

Short-term problems

If the posterior surface of the contact lens is too flat, it will move excessively on the cornea and the edge of the lens may cross the visual axis and cause the vision to fluctuate with each blink. Movement of the upper eyelid during blinking over a soft contact lens presses it against the cornea and causes a temporary fluctuation in the visual acuity.

The quoted power of a soft contact lens denotes its power when it is suspended in saline at room temperature. Small changes occur when the lens is in use: the lens moulds to the surface curvature of the cornea, the evaporation of water increases the refractive index and an increase in temperature increases the curvature (the latter two factors increase the negative power of the lens). The dry atmosphere of an aircraft cabin may cause blurred vision during and after a flight because of the increased evaporation of water from soft contact lenses.

Long-term problems

Corneal warpage is the change in corneal curvature induced by wearing a contact lens which is not associated with corneal oedema. It regresses after the lens is removed over hours or days. During this time, any spectacles which were once accurate no longer compensate for the altered shape of the cornea and spectacle blur results. Warpage is more pronounced and of longer duration when more rigid lenses are worn. It is important not to perform refractive surgery or biometry (to estimate intraocular lens power) or to prescribe spectacles before these changes have stabilised.

13   Optics of Low Vision Aids

Magnifying devices of several kinds are in wide use to assist the poorly sighted patient in daily life. Most so-called 'low vision aids' are designed to be used as reading aids, that is, for near vision. However, other devices exist to assist distance vision, e.g. to enable the patient to read bus numbers and watch television. In this chapter, the underlying optical principles of low vision aids are described.

For a fuller account of the different forms available and their clinical application the reader is recommended to read the literature on the subject.

All low vision aids work by presenting the patient with a magnified view of the object. Most are optical systems which act by increasing the angle subtended by the object at the eye, thus producing an enlarged retinal image (cf. angular magnification, p. 60). The magnifying power (MP) of such an optical system can be defined as

$$MP = \frac{\text{retinal image size with use of instrument}}{\text{retinal image size without use of instrument}}$$

Projection systems are also coming into use as low vision aids. An enlarged image of the object is presented to the patient on a screen which he or she can view from a convenient distance. Closed circuit television is one means of achieving this and is in limited use.

The basic optics of the optical systems used as low vision aids (LVA) is described below.

The convex lens

The use of the convex lens as a magnifying loupe was described in Chapter 5. A high-power simple convex lens mounted in a spectacle frame works in the same way. The magnifying power is achieved by allowing the eye to view the object at closer range than would be possible unaided or with a standard presbyopic reading correction. However, the power of lens used, e.g. +5.0 DS, is less than that of the standard loupe (× 8 = +32 DS) so that in this case the convex lens may be regarded as an enhanced presbyopic correction (Fig. 13.1). Convex lenses are also used as hand-held magnifiers, or mounted on legs as 'stand magnifiers'. The object is located between the first principal focus and the lens, and a magnified virtual image is produced which is viewed by

a Object viewed at 40 cm with standard +2.50 DS presbyopic correction

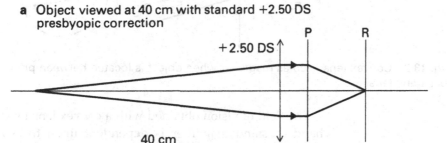

b Object viewed at 20 cm with + 5.0 DS convex lens

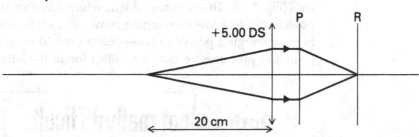

c Angle subtended at eye by object at 40 cm compared with angle subtended at eye by object at 20 cm

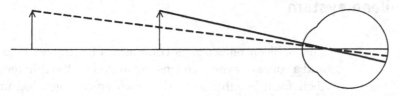

Fig. 13.1 Convex spectacle lens as LVA. Example: a 65-year old emmetrope with age-related macular degeneration (P = principal plane, R = retina).

the eye. As the object moves nearer to the first principal focus, F_1 (Fig. 13.2), the virtual image becomes larger and is situated further from the eye. Thus a hand-held magnifier can be positioned by the user so that the image is formed at a comfortable viewing distance from the eye. Stand magnifiers are made so that the optimum object-lens distance is maintained. A variant is the 'paper weight' plano-convex lens which is very thick and rests directly on the page.

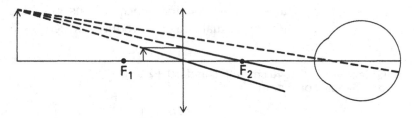

Fig. 13.2 Convex lens used as magnifier when object is located between principal focus and lens.

The field of vision obtained with a convex lens used as a hand or stand magnifier is dependent upon the size or aperture of the lens, and on the eye-lens distance. The greater the eye-lens distance, the smaller the field of vision.

Convex cylindrical lenses are also employed as reading aids (Fig. 13.3). The bar-shaped lens which has no refractive power or only a low converging power in its long axis and high converging power in cross-section is laid on a line of print and produces vertical magnification of the letters.

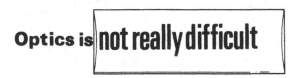

Fig. 13.3 Convex cylindrical magnifying lens.

The Galilean system

The Galilean telescope is composed of a convex objective and a concave eye-piece lens, separated by the difference of their focal lengths. It produces an erect magnified image and the image is not greatly distorted by curvature of field or astigmatism (cf. Chapter 8). Furthermore, the system is compact and light and thus very suitable for use as a magnifying aid – usually mounted in a spectacle frame. It can be adapted for viewing near or distant objects but it is difficult to combine near and distance use in the same instrument.

The Galilean telescope (Fig. 13.4) magnifies by increasing the angle subtended by the object at the eye.

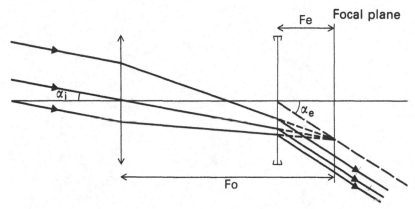

Fig. 13.4 Galilean telescope.

$$\text{Angular magnification, } M = \frac{\alpha_e}{\alpha_i}$$

where α_e is the angle of emergence, and α_i is the angle of incidence.

It can be shown mathematically that

$$M = \frac{Fe}{Fo}$$

where Fe is the power of the eye-piece lens in dioptres, and Fo is the power of the objective lens in dioptres.

The practical usefulness of optical magnifying devices as low vision aids is limited by the following factors.

(1) High magnification results in a reduced field of view, which makes rapid scanning of a line or page of print impossible. This factor also limits the usefulness of a distance low vision aid.

(2) The object to be viewed has to be held close to the eye.

(3) Magnification means that depth of focus is reduced. Thus the object–lens distance is critical.

In practice, any unsteadiness of hand or head leads to unpleasant instability of field and focus.

Therefore, the aim of the prescriber should be to provide the lowest magnification that is adequate for the patient's requirements in a useable and acceptable form.

14 Instruments

Direct ophthalmoscope

The direct ophthalmoscope is commonly used for routine examination of the fundus of the eye, especially when a slit lamp cannot be used. It is small, easily portable and can also be used to examine the more anterior parts of the eye. It is important, therefore, to understand how it works, and its advantages and limitations.

The instrument consists of a system of lenses which focus light from an electric bulb on to a mirror where a real image of the bulb filament is formed. The mirror reflects the emitted light in a diverging beam which is used to illuminate the patient's eye. The mirror contains a hole through which the observer views the illuminated eye. The image of the bulb is formed just below the hole so that its corneal reflection does not lie in the visual axis of the observer (Fig. 14.1).

The area of retina which can be seen at any one time is called the field of view. It is governed by the projected image of the sight-hole on the retina (the sight-hole being the hole in the mirror or the observer's pupil, whichever is the smaller). The image A^1B^1 of the sight-hole AB is constructed (Fig. 14.2) using a ray through the nodal point, N, and a ray parallel to the visual axis which is refracted by the eye to pass through its posterior focal point.

Figure 14.3 shows the area of retina on to which image A^1B^1 is projected, which is the field of view. The figure shows that the field of view is smaller in a myopic eye, R_m, and larger in a hypermetropic eye, R_h, than in an emmetropic eye, R.

Figure 14.4 shows that the field of view is considerably

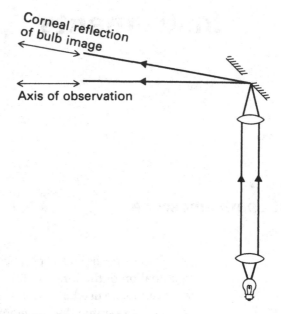

Fig. 14.1   The direct ophthalmoscope.

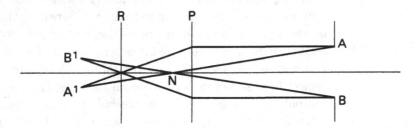

Fig. 14.2   Direct ophthalmoscope. Image of sight-hole formed by emmetropic eye. R = retina; P = principal plane.

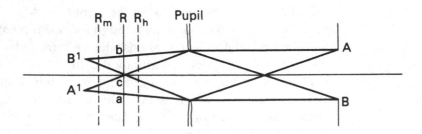

Fig. 14.3   Direct ophthalmoscope. Field of view ab (projected image of sight-hole on retina of emmetropic eye, R, myopic eye R_m and hypermetropic eye R_h).

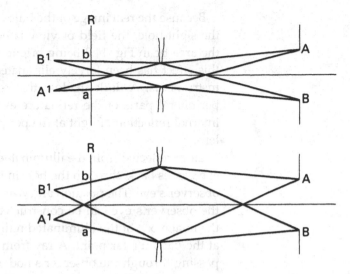

Fig. 14.4 Direct ophthalmoscope. Effect of pupil size on field of view ab.

enlarged when the pupil is dilated; hence the advantage of instilling a mydriatic prior to fundoscopy.

In order to utilise the maximum available field of view it is necessary for the observer to be as close as possible to the patient's eye. Figure 14.5 shows that as the distance between the patient and the observer decreases, the field of view (the projected image of the sight-hole on the patient's retina) becomes larger.

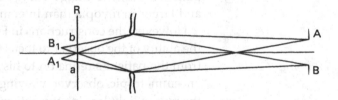

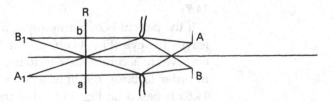

Fig. 14.5 Direct ophthalmoscope. The field of view ab increases as the sight-hole approaches the patient's eye.

Because the real image of the bulb filament lies just below the sight-hole, the field of view is not evenly illuminated, the area bc in Fig. 14.3 being brighter than the area ac, but this effect has been largely eliminated in the most modern instruments. A dark shadow that is often seen when the peripheral parts of the retina are examined is due to total internal reflection of light at the periphery of the crystalline lens.

Light reflected from the illuminated retina of the patient's eye passes back, through the hole in the mirror and into the observer's eye. The position and size of the image formed in the observer's eye can be constructed by first constructing the image, xy, of the illuminated retina XY which is formed at the patient's far point. A ray from the top of that image, passing through the observer's nodal point, N_o, locates the position of the top of the image, X'Y', on the observer's retina R_o. (If this construction is used, it is not necessary for the patient's and observer's anterior focal points to coincide – a condition rarely fulfilled in practice.) In Figs 14.6, 14.7 and 14.8, R, P, N and F_a are the patient's retina, principal plane, nodal point and anterior focal point respectively, while R_o, P_o and N_o refer to the observer's retina, principal plane and nodal point.

It can be seen from Fig. 14.6 that the image formed in the observer's eye is inverted and is therefore seen as erect. Also, the image size varies with the refractive state of the patient's eye, the image being smaller in hypermetropia, and larger in myopia than in emmetropia.

However, the constructions in Fig. 14.6 take no account of the ability of the observer to focus the beam of light reflected from the patient's retina on to his own retina. In the case of an emmetropic observer viewing an emmetropic patient, the rays of light leaving the patient's eye are parallel and are therefore focused on the observer's retina without any accommodative effort or the use of a correcting lens (Fig. 14.7).

If the patient is hypermetropic, a diverging beam of light leaves his eye (Fig. 14.6b) and it behoves an emmetropic observer to accommodate or to use a correcting convex lens in order to bring the light to a focus on his retina. Figure 14.8a is based on Fig. 14.6b, but the pencil of light around the ray which passes through N_o, the observer's nodal point, has been added to show that the point X' (and Y') in

a Emmetropic patient

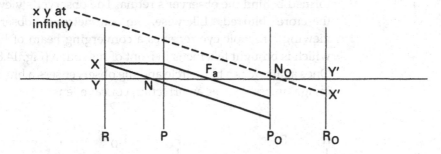

b Hypermetropic patient

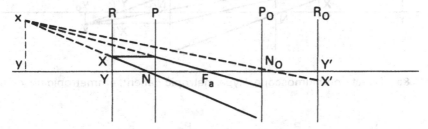

c Myopic patient

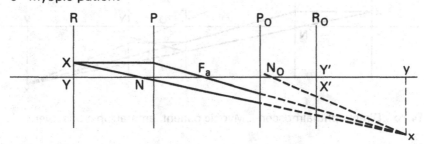

Fig. 14.6 Direct ophthalmoscope. Construction of image in observer's eye.

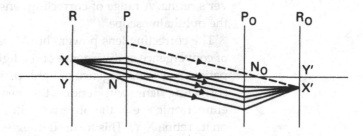

Fig. 14.7 Direct ophthalmoscope. Emmetropic patient and observer.

Fig. 14.6b is really a blur circle as a virtual image $x_o y_o$ is formed behind the observer's retina. The observer's view is therefore blurred. Likewise, an emmetropic observer viewing a myopic eye receives a converging beam of light which is brought to a focus in front of his retina (Fig. 14.8b). Once again, X' is a blur circle and the observer sees a blurred image unless he uses a correcting concave lens.

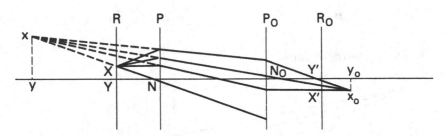

Fig. 14.8a Direct ophthalmoscope. Hypermetropic patient, emmetropic observer.

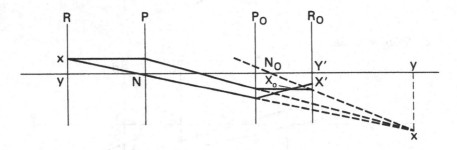

Fig. 14.8b Direct ophthalmoscope. Myopic patient, emmetropic observer.

In order to see a clear view of the patient's retina in myopia or hypermetropia, it is therefore necessary to use a correcting lens to bring the image to a focus on the observer's retina. A range of correcting lenses is incorporated in the ophthalmoscope.

The correcting lens power should be equal to the degree of convergence or divergence of the light emerging from the patient's eye (cf. vergence of light, p. 59, Fig. 5.8). Thus, the correcting lens will render the beam parallel and the emmetropic eye of the observer will form a focused image on its retina $X_r Y_r$. This focused image can be constructed by drawing the emerging light and image xy of XY formed at the patient's far point as before (cf. Fig. 14.6). A ray from x, passing through the centre of the correcting lens, determines the direction of the parallel beam formed after refraction of the emerging beam by the correcting lens. The ray in the parallel beam which passes through the observer's nodal point N_o locates X_r on the retina (Fig. 14.9).

(a) Emmetropic patient

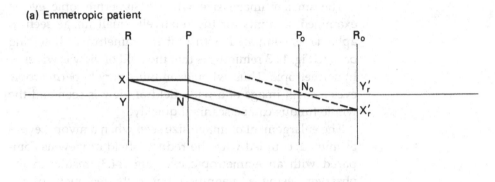

(b) Hypermetropic patient

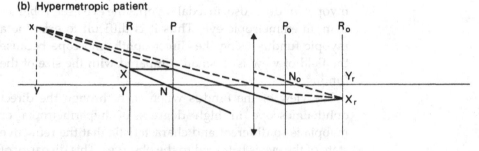

(c) Myopic patient

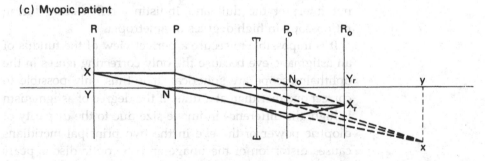

Fig. 14.9 Direct ophthalmoscope. Construction of image in observer's eye when a correcting lens is used.

The image formed on the observer's retina is smaller when a hypermetropic eye is viewed and larger when a myopic eye is viewed than when an emmetropic eye is examined, but the use of a correcting lens reduces the discrepancy in size (Fig. 14.9). (If the patient's and the observer's anterior focal points coincide, and the correcting lens is placed at that point, the observer's image is the same size regardless of whether the patient is hypermetropic, emmetropic or myopic. However, these conditions are rarely fulfilled in practice.)

The smaller image size when a hypermetropic eye is examined accounts for the relatively small image seen in aphakia as compared with that in emmetropia. Referring back to Fig. 14.3 reminds us that the field of view is wider in hypermetropia. Thus, when examining very hypermetropic eyes a small image of a wide field of view is seen and the whole fundus can be scanned quickly.

The enlargement of image size seen when a myopic eye is examined, coupled with the reduced field of view as compared with an emmetropic eye (Fig. 14.3) results in the observer seeing a magnified but restricted view of the myopic fundus. Also, in axial myopia the eye itself is bigger than an emmetropic eye. Thus it is difficult to examine a myopic fundus using the direct ophthalmoscope because the field of view is so small compared with the size of the fundus.

The view of the fundus when seen through the direct ophthalmoscope in high degrees of hypermetropia or myopia is so different and characteristic that the refractive state of the eye is betrayed to the observer. This disparity of appearance can be made use of when the refractionist cannot interpret the dull and indistinct reflex seen during retinoscopy in high degrees of ametropia.

It is impossible to secure a perfect view of the fundus of an astigmatic eye because the only correcting lenses in the ophthalmoscope are spherical. It is thus only possible to correct one meridian at a time. If the degree of astigmatism is high, the difference in image size due to the disparity of dioptric power of the eye in the two principal meridians causes distortion of the image and the optic disc appears oval.

Thus far it has been assumed that the observer is emmetropic. For those observers who have a refractive error there are two possibilities. The observer can remove his spectacles and rack up the appropriate lens in the ophthalmoscope to give a clear view of the patient's fundus. The appropriate lens is the algebraic sum of his own and the patient's refractive error (the value is approximate because the position of the correcting lens influences its effectivity [see p. 121]). Alternatively, he can use the instrument with his glasses on. However, his field of view will be restricted as the sight-hole in the mirror will be further from his eye.

The patient's refractive error can be roughly judged by noting the power of the correcting lens used. This, however, assumes that neither patient nor observer is accommodating.

The posterior pole of a highly myopic fundus is best seen with the direct ophthalmoscope if the patient keeps his glasses on. The magnification of the patient's retina when viewed through the direct ophthalmoscope may be calculated. The underlying principle is the same as that of the loupe (Chapter 5). The observer is using the dioptric power of the patient's eye as a loupe and is thus able to inspect the patient's retina at close quarters, i.e. well within his near point of distinct vision, and yet see it clearly.

The formula for magnification achieved by a loupe is $M = F/4$ where M is the magnification and F the dioptric power of the loupe. If we ascribe a dioptric power of $+60\,D$ to the patient's emmetropic eye, the magnification of the direct ophthalmoscope is $\times 15$. This degree of magnification makes the direct ophthalomoscope particularly useful when examining patients with retinopathy, for it allows most micro-aneurysms to be seen. However, some are too small to be visualised with this instrument. Many modern direct ophthalmoscopes incorporate a red-free filter. The resulting green light causes the micro-aneurysms to show up as black dots against a green background and this makes their detection easier.

The direct ophthalmoscope can also be used as a self-illuminating loupe to examine the anterior segment of the eye, e.g. lens opacities can be directly inspected through the $+10\,D$ correcting lens.

Indirect ophthalmoscope

The indirect ophthalmoscope offers an alternative means of examining the retina and vitreous, and gives a very different view of the retina compared with that obtained with the direct ophthalmoscope. Both instruments have their place and should be used to complement each other during the clinical examination of the eye. Table 14.1 sets out the characteristics of the two instruments.

Table 14.1 Summary of the optical properties of the direct and indirect ophthalmoscope.

	Direct ophthalmoscope	Indirect ophthalmoscope
Image	Not inverted	Vertically and horizontally inverted
Field of view	Small (6°)	Large (25°)
Magnification	Large (× 15)	Small (× 3 [+20 D]) (× 5 [+13 D])
Binocularity	Not available	Stereoscopic view
Influence of patient's refractive error	Large	Small
Teaching facility	None	Teaching mirror (Fig. 3.5 and text)

In the indirect method of ophthalmoscopy a powerful convex lens (hereafter called the condensing lens) is held in front of the patient's eye. The usual powers used are +20 D and +13 D. The illuminating light beam passes through the condensing lens into the eye and light reflected from the retina is refracted by the condensing lens to form a real image between the condensing lens and the observer. The observer studies this real image of the patient's retina (Fig. 14.10).

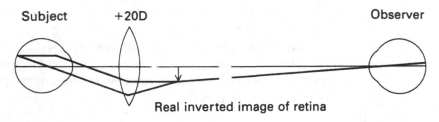

Subject   +20D   Observer

Real inverted image of retina

Fig. 14.10   Indirect ophthalmoscope.

Illumination is usually provided by an electric lamp mounted on the observer's head. Light from this source is rendered convergent by the condensing lens. Thus a convergent beam enters the patient's eye and is brought to a focus within the vitreous by the eye's refractive system.

The light then diverges to strike the retina (Fig. 14.11). The illumination is therefore bright and even, as it comes from the real image of the light source within the patient's eye.

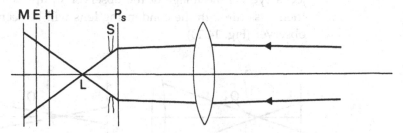

Fig. 14.11 Indirect ophthalmoscope. Field of illumination.

Figure 14.11 illustrates the path of the illuminating beam, P_s being the subject's principal plane, S his pupil and M, E and H being the retina in myopia, emmetropia and hypermetropia respectively. The diagram shows that the field of illumination is largest in myopia and smallest in hypermetropia and that in all refractive states the size of the subject's pupil limits the field of illumination.

The condensing lens is held in front of the patient's eye at such a distance that the patient's pupil and the observer's pupil are conjugate foci. (This means that light arising from a point in the subject's pupillary plane is brought to a focus by the condensing lens in the observer's pupillary plane, and vice versa.) A reduced image of the observer's pupil is therefore formed in the subject's pupillary plane (Fig. 14.12) (the image of a 4 mm pupil is approximately 0.7 mm). Only those rays of light which leave the subject's eye via the area of the image of the observer's pupil can, after refraction by the condensing lens, enter the observer's pupil and be seen

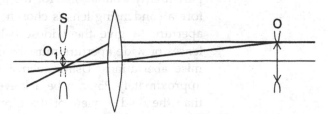

Fig. 14.12 Indirect ophthalmoscope. Construction of the reduced image O_1 of the observer's pupil O in the subject's pupillary plane S.

by him. The observer's pupil is the 'sight-hole' of the system and its size influences the field of view.

The field of view is also limited by the aperture or size of the condensing lens. Only those rays which leave the subject's eye via the image of the observer's pupil and which then pass through the condensing lens will be seen by the observer (Fig. 14.13).

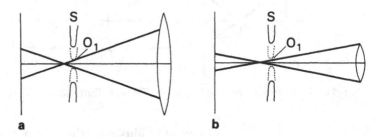

Fig. 14.13 Indirect ophthalmoscope. The field of view is limited by the image of the observer's pupil O_1 in the subject's pupil S and by the aperture of the condensing lens. (a) When a large aperture condensing lens is used, the field of view is limited only by the observer's pupil O_1. (b) When a small aperture condensing lens is used, it is the lens aperture that limits the field of view.

Thus, to recap, the subject's pupil size determines the field of illumination, Fig. 14.11. The observer's pupil size and the aperture of the condensing lens determine the field of view (Figs. 14.13a and b).

It is usual to dilate the patient's pupil widely prior to indirect ophthalmoscopic examination, in order to widen the field of illumination. It is not practical to dilate the observer's pupil because his visual acuity would be impaired. This is because he would suffer an increase in aberrations and loss of accommodation, the latter being particularly troublesome for the low hypermetrope. Therefore a condensing lens is chosen with the largest possible aperture to give the widest field of view. Condensing lenses of wide aperture must be of aspheric form to minimise aberrations. Using such a lens, a field of view of approximately 25° can be achieved, i.e. four times larger than the field of view of the direct ophthalmoscope. This is a great advantage when a highly myopic eye is to be examined.

Light emerging from the patient's eye is refracted by the

condensing lens to form a real image of the retina between the condensing lens and the observer. The image is both vertically and laterally inverted (upside down and back to front). It is situated at or near the second principal focus of the condensing lens, i.e. approximately 8 cm in front of a +13 D lens (Fig. 14.14). The observer holds the condensing lens at arm's length and thus views the image from a distance of 40–50 cm. Therefore, to see the image clearly the observer must accommodate or use a presbyopic correction. The binocular indirect opthalmoscopes have +2.0 D lenses incorporated in the binocular prismatic eyepieces so that the observer does not need to accommodate. (However, those observers whose near correction is more than +2.0 DS because of underlying hypermetropia, or who have any significant refractive error, need to wear their spectacle correction when using the instrument.)

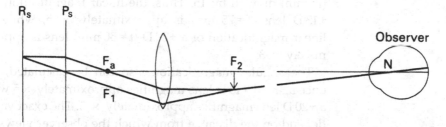

Fig. 14.14 Indirect ophthalmoscope. Formation of the real image of the subject's retina. The image is viewed by the observer (image-observer distance foreshortened).

The linear magnification of the image can be calculated from Fig. 14.15. Parallel light emerges from the retina AB of the emmetropic subject's eye, and is refracted by the condensing lens to form an image ab in its principal focal plane F.

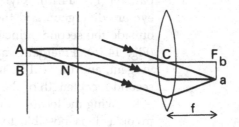

Fig. 14.15 Indirect ophthalmoscope. Linear magnification.

$$\text{Linear magnification} = \frac{ab}{AB}$$

However, angle aCF = angle ANB because Ca and AN are parallel.

$$\text{Tan aCF} = \frac{ab}{CF} = \text{tan ANB} = \frac{AB}{BN}$$

Therefore

$$\frac{ab}{AB} = \frac{CF}{BN}$$

CF is the focal length of the condensing lens. BN is the distance between the nodal point and the retina of the subject's eye. If this distance BN is taken to be 15 mm, the linear magnification is equal to the focal length of the lens (in mm) divided by 15. Thus, the linear magnification of a +13 D lens (f = 75 mm) is approximately × 5, while the linear magnification of a +20 D (f = 50 mm) lens is approximately × 3.

The angular magnification also can be calculated, and once again a +13 D lens magnifies approximately × 5 while a +20 D lens magnifies approximately × 3. The exact values depend on the distance from which the observer views the real image of the subject's retina, and upon the distance between the condensing lens and the subject's eye if this is ametropic (see below).

The refractive state of the patient's eye affects the size and position of the real image formed by the condensing lens.

The image of the retina of an emmetropic eye is always located at the second principal focus of the condensing lens, regardless of the position of the lens relative to the eye. This is because all rays emerging from an emmetropic eye are parallel (Fig. 14.15). Rays emerging from a hypermetropic eye are divergent, and the real image is therefore formed outside the second principal focus of the condensing lens (Fig. 14.16). Emergent rays from a myopic eye are convergent, and the real image is therefore always within the second focal length of the lens.

Knowing the location of the image in hypermetropia and myopia, it is possible to study the effect of moving the condensing lens relative to the eye.

Figure 14.17 shows the changes in image size when the

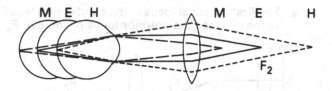

Fig. 14.16 Indirect ophthalmoscope. Relative positions of the image in hypermetropia H, emmetropia, E, and myopia, M.

first principal focus of the condensing lens F_1 is moved relative to the anterior focus F_a of the eye. A ray parallel to the optical axis of the eye which, after refraction at the principal plane, passes through F_a is used to determine the relative image sizes in hypemetropia, emmetropia and myopia.

The image size in emmetropia is the same in all positions of the condensing lens, and is determined by a ray through F_1 (dotted) parallel to the emergent ray through F_a, which after refraction by the condensing lens is parallel to the principal axis of the lens.

In myopia, the image size increases as the condensing lens is moved away from the eye, while in hypermetropia the image becomes smaller. This effect can be used by the examiner to assess the refractive condition of the subject's eye.

The relative merits of the direct and indirect ophthalmoscope

Other considerations include:

(1) Size of the instrument. The direct ophthalmoscope is much smaller and lighter than the indirect, and many models are pocket size.

(2) Illumination is crucial to the view obtained. Because indirect ophthalmoscopes are larger instruments, there is more scope for fitting more powerful light sources. This renders the indirect ophthalmoscope more useful in examining patients with opacities in the ocular media.

(3) The combination of good illumination and wide field of view makes the indirect ophthalmoscope the

a The first principal focus of the condensing lens F₁ is closer
to the eye than the anterior focus of the eye Fₐ

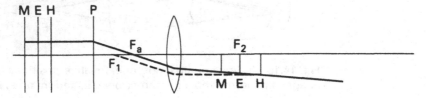

b The first principal focus of the condensing lens F₁ is at the
anterior focus of the eye Fₐ

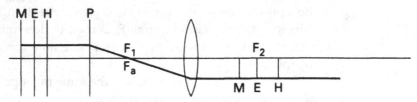

c The first principal focus of the condensing lens F₁ is beyond
the anterior focus of the eye Fₐ

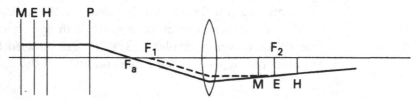

Fig. 14.17 Indirect ophthalmoscope. To show the effect on image size of moving the condensing lens progressively further away from the subject's eye in ametropia.

instrument of choice when examining patients with retinal detachments. If there is extensive subretinal fluid and the illumination is poor, an underlying malignancy may not be seen with the direct ophthalmoscope. Furthermore, examination with the indirect ophthalmoscope also allows identation of the peripheral retina.

(4) The indirect ophthalmoscope is also the ophthalmoscope of choice for use during retinal detachment surgery because it is used at a distance which allows the surgeon to preserve a sterile operative field.

(5) Laser energy can be delivered through the indirect ophthalmoscope to effect retinal photocoagulation.

Retinoscope

An accurate objective measurement of the refractive state of an eye can be made using the retinoscope. The technique is called *retinoscopy*.

Light is directed into the patient's eye to illuminate the retina (the illumination stage). An image of the illuminated retina is formed at the patient's far-point (the reflex stage). The image at the far-point is located by moving the illumination across the fundus and noting the behaviour of the luminous reflex seen by the observer in the patient's pupil (the projection stage).

Illumination stage

Figures 14.18 and 14.19a and b illustrate the simple system of illumination that was used before hand-held electric retinoscopes came into use. A light source was located beside the patient's head, and light reflected into the patient's eye from a plane or concave mirror held by the observer. The observer viewed the patient's eye through a small hole in the mirror. The electric retinoscope has largely replaced this system. However, the principles and nomenclature have remained unchanged.

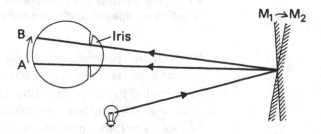

Fig. 14.18 Illumination stage. Plane mirror.

When a plane mirror is used, light is moved across the patient's fundus from A to B by rotating the plane mirror from M_1 to M_2. Note that the illuminating rays move in the same direction as the mirror.

A concave mirror of focal length less than the distance between patient and observer is occasionally used for retinoscopy. A real image of the light source is formed

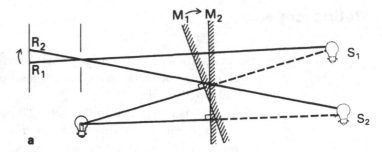

Fig. 14.19a   Illumination stage. Plane mirror. Virtual images S_1 and S_2 of light source S (located by their normals to the mirror [see Chapter 2]) throw light via the nodal point so that the movement of illumination at the retina, R_1 to R_2, is 'with' the movement of the mirror, M_1 to M_2.

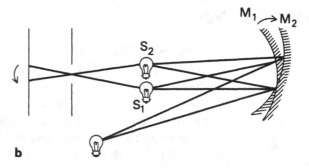

Fig. 14.19b   Illumination stage. Concave mirror. Real images S_1 and S_2 of the light source throw the light via the nodal point so that the illumination at the retina moves in the opposite direction or 'against' the movement of the mirror, M_1 to M_2.

between the patient and the observer, and close to the patient's eye. This real image acts as a bright light source for illuminating the patient's retina. However, the illumination moves in the opposite direction to the mirror (see Fig. 14.19b). Thus the movement of the reflex seen by the observer is reversed compared with the plane mirror. The modern electric retinoscope incorporates both these systems of illumination. This is achieved by the use of a condensing lens which can be moved within the shaft of the instrument. At its lowest position the plane mirror effect is obtained and at its highest position the effect is that of the concave mirror.

If the condensing lens is moved from the lowest (plane mirror) position upwards along the shaft of the instrument, an intermediate position is reached at which a focused image of the retinoscope bulb filament falls on the patient's eye (or cheek). The effect is that of a concave mirror of focal length equalling the retinoscope–patient distance and is of no value for retinoscopy as the image of the light source is coincident with the patient's eye. However, if the retinoscope condensing lens is moved a short distance back down the shaft of the retinoscope, the 'plane mirror effect' is regained but with a much brighter illumination than that obtained with the condensing lens at its lowest position. This is because a virtual image S_1 of the light source is formed just behind the patient's eye (Fig. 14.20). The retinoscope is now acting as a concave mirror of focal length slightly exceeding the observer–patient distance.

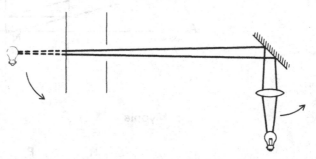

Fig. 14.20 Electric retinoscope adjusted for use as concave mirror of focal length slightly exceeding the observer–patient distance, thus obtaining plane mirror effect. The whole instrument is tilted to achieve movement of the illumination across the patient's retina (arrows).

This arrangement is useful in clinical practice for two reasons. First, the plane mirror effect (which most observers prefer) is retained. And, secondly, a bright light is achieved which makes retinoscopy easier when the pupil is small and when there are opacities in the media of the eye.

Reflex stage

Because the plane mirror effect is usually preferred in retinoscopy, the following description and diagrams illustrate the plane mirror effect.

An image A_1B_1 of the illuminated retina is formed at the patient's far-point (pp. 109, 118). This image may be constructed using three rays (Fig. 14.21).

a Hypermetropia

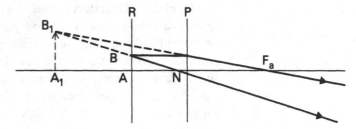

b Emmetropia

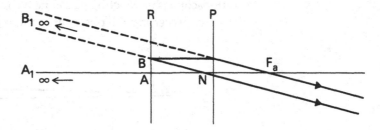

c Myopia

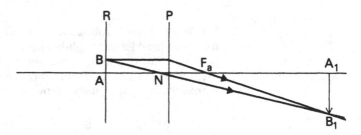

Fig. 14.21 Reflex stage of retinoscopy.

(1)   A ray from point A of the retina R on the principal axis of the eye, which leaves the eye along the principal axis.

(2)   A ray from a retinal point B, off the principal axis, which travels parallel to the principal axis as far as the principal plane, P, of the eye, where it is refracted to pass onward through the anterior principal focus, F_a, of the eye.

(3)   A ray from retinal point B which passes undeviated through the nodal point, N.

(NB When drawing these diagrams from memory, construct the image at the far-point for each refractive condition and

F_a will look after itself. Do not put F_a at a random position and then try to make the diagram 'work'.)

Projection stage

The observer views the image A_1B_1 of the illuminated retina AB from a convenient distance, usually $\frac{2}{3}$ m. Figure 14.22 depicts this and is constructed by drawing Fig. 14.21 and adding a hypothetical ray from point B_1 passing through the observer's nodal point, N_o, to the observer's retina, R_o. This ray locates the point B_o, the image of B_1 on the observer's retina, and allows completion of the diagram. The observer does not see the actual image A_1B_1, but rays from A_1B_1 are seen as an illuminated area or reflex in the patient's pupil.

In hypermetropia the luminous reflex seen in the patient's pupil moves in the same direction as the illuminating light – a 'with' movement, indicated by the arrows in Fig. 14.22. Once again a 'with' movement is observed.

When the patient's myopia is less than the dioptric value of the observer's working distance a 'with' movement is still obtained.

Figures 14.22a–c illustrate that the angle $A_oN_oB_o$ increases progressively as a refractive error equal to the dioptric value

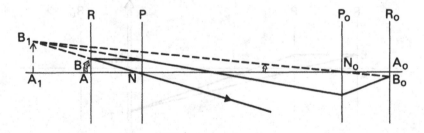

Fig. 14.22a Projection stage. Hypermetropia.

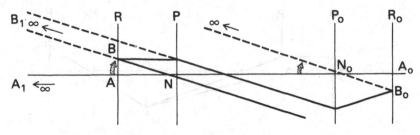

Fig. 14.22b Projection stage. Emmetropia.

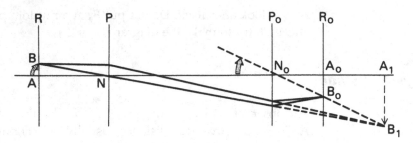

Fig. 14.22c Projection stage. Myopia less than −1.5 D (for working distance of $\frac{2}{3}$ metre).

of the observer's working distance (1.5 D) is approached. Therefore the luminous reflex appears to move more rapidly as this point is approached. The *point of reversal* or *neutral point* of retinoscopy is reached when the patient's far-point coincides with the observer's nodal point (Fig. 14.22d). No image of B_1 can be formed on the observer's retina and at this point no movement of the reflex can be discerned in the patient's pupil. The observer sees a diffuse bright red reflex. This is because the movement of the reflex is infinitely rapid.

When the patient's myopia exceeds the dioptric value of the working distance, the image A_1B_1 falls between the

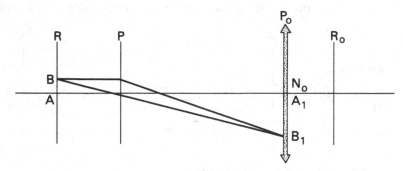

Fig. 14.22d Projection stage. Point of reversal.

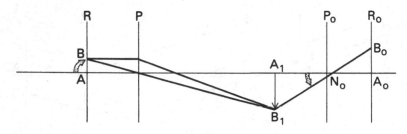

Fig. 14.22e Projection stage. Myopia greater than −1.5 D (for working distance of $\frac{2}{3}$ metre).

patient and the observer. The diagram shows that the luminous reflex now appears to move in the opposite direction to the illuminating light; 'against' movement. Once again the luminous reflex appears to move more rapidly as the point of reversal is approached.

In practice, lenses are placed in front of the patient's eye until the point of reversal is seen by the observer. A correction is made for the working distance (add –1.5 D for $\frac{2}{3}$ m, add –1.0 D for 1 m) and the corrected value of the lenses equals the patient's refractive error. A full discussion of practical retinoscopy will be found in Chapter 15. Automated refraction is discussed in Chapter 16.

Instruments used to study corneal curvature

The anterior corneal surface is the main refracting surface of the eye (p. 105). Its curvature is crucial to the refracting power and optical properties of the eye. A small change in curvature or irregularity of the corneal surface has a profound effect upon visual acuity.

Accurate measurement of the corneal curvature is important in ophthalmology and indeed essential in contact lens fitting.

The anterior corneal surface reflects a small portion of any light incident upon it and thus acts as a convex mirror. The corneal surface and curvature can be examined by studying the catoptric image so formed (see p. 111).

Placido's disc

The general shape of the cornea can be studied using Placido's disc. This is a flat disc bearing concentric black and white rings (Fig. 14.23). A convex lens is mounted in an aperture in the centre of the disc in order to magnify the image and relieve the need for accommodation. The examiner looks through the central aperture and observes the image of the disc formed by reflection from the patient's cornea. (Best results are obtained by ensuring that the disc is brightly illuminated by adjusting the light behind the patient's head leaving the patient's eye in shadow.)

The nature of the image seen betrays the regularity or distortion of corneal curvature to the examiner. The shorter

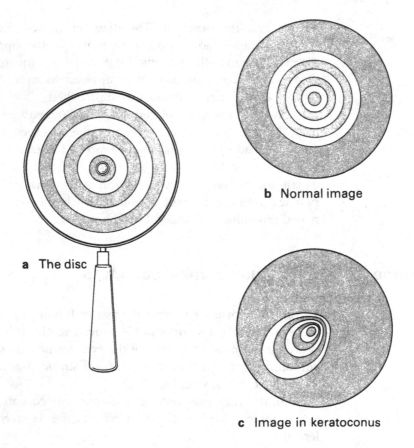

a   The disc

b   Normal image

c   Image in keratoconus

Fig. 14.23   Placido's disc.

the radius of curvature of the anterior surface of the cornea, the smaller the reflected image and the closer the reflected rings of the Placido disc lie to one another. When viewing an astigmatic cornea, the rings appear closer in the steeper meridian.

The same principle may be used during surgery to detect the presence of corneal astigmatism and to guide corneal suturing. The surgeon observes the regularity of the corneal reflection from a circular object by looking through the centre of, for example, a ring of lights or a hollow cone with rings along the inner surface.

Keratometer or ophthalmometer

The radius of curvature of the central area of the cornea can be measured using a keratometer (sometimes called an ophthalmometer). Two main types are available but both measure the radius of curvature of a central zone of the cornea approximately 3 mm in diameter.

The central or axial area of the cornea, about 4 mm in diameter, is usually assumed to be a spherical refracting surface. The keratometer thus reads within this zone. The radius of curvature of the axial zone of the emmetropic eye is about 7.8 mm. The optical power of the cornea can also be expressed in dioptres. The precise value is determined by the curvature of the anterior and posterior surfaces as well as the refractive indices of the cornea and the media at each surface. However, for most corneas an approximation is provided by the keratometer equation in which the refractive index of tears (1.336) is standardized to 1.3375 so that a radius of curvature of 7.5 mm corresponds to 45D (cf. p. 36):

$$D = \frac{n_2 - n_1}{r} = \frac{1.3375 - 1}{r}$$

where D is the power in dioptres and r is the radius of the anterior corneal curvature expressed in metres. For example,

$$D = \frac{1.3375 - 1}{0.0078} = +43.27 \text{ D}$$

The more peripheral cornea is flatter and non-spherical. Optically, it is the central 4 mm spherical zone which is utilised for vision, the periphery being screened off by the pupil. Visual acuity suffers when the pupil is widely dilated.

The principle on which the keratometer works is now explained (Fig. 14.24).

$$\frac{I}{O} = \frac{v}{u}$$

In practice, I is located very close to F/ therefore v may be taken to equal r/2 where r is the radius of curvature of the reflecting surface. Substituting,

$$\frac{I}{O} = \frac{v}{u} = \frac{r}{2u}$$

$$r = 2u \times \frac{I}{O}$$

In all keratometers u is constant, being the focal distance of the viewing telescope. The von Helmholtz keratometer

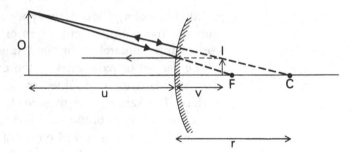

Fig. 14.24 Keratometer. Underlying optical principle.

has a fixed object size and the image size is adjusted to measure the corneal curvature, while in the Javal Schiøtz instrument the object size is varied to achieve a standard image size.

In order to study closely and measure the image formed by reflection at the cornea, some means must be adopted to overcome the natural movements of the patient's eye. Even small movements cause the image to 'dance about'.

This difficulty has been overcome by doubling the image seen by the examiner. Thus if the patient's eye moves, both images move together and a reading can be made by aligning the images one with the other.

The keratometer of von Helmholtz

The von Helmholtz keratometer uses two rotating glass plates to achieve doubling of the image. A beam of light which has passed through a graticule is shone on to the patient's cornea where an image I of the graticule is formed by reflection. The reflected light passes back into the instrument through two parallel-sided glass plates X and Y which are inclined to each other. These plates displace the light laterally as it passes through them, thus giving rise to two virtual images of I, I' and I" which are viewed through a telescope (Fig. 14.25). The angle of inclination of the glass plates is varied by the observer until the edges of I' and I" touch. The distance between their centres then equals the diameter of I, from which the corneal curvature can be calculated. In fact, the instrument is calibrated in terms of corneal radius of curvature and of dioptric power of the cornea.

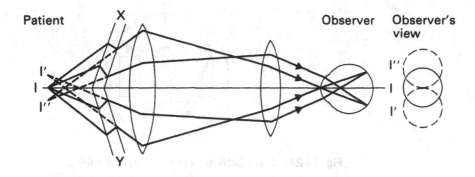

Fig. 14.25 Von Helmholtz keratometer and measurement of corneal curvature.

The instrument can be rotated to allow measurement of astigmatism in a similar manner to the Javal–Schiøtz keratometer.

The Javal–Schiøtz keratometer

The Javal–Schiøtz keratometer uses an object of variable size. The object consists of a pair of mires, A and B, mounted on curved side arms which project each side of the viewing telescope (Fig. 14.26). Each mire consists of a small lantern with a coloured window. One mire is step shaped while the other is rectangular. The *space between the mires ab* is the object size used in the measurement (Fig. 14.27). The arms

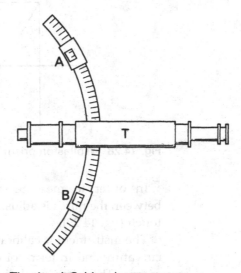

Fig. 14.26 The Javal–Schiøtz keratometer.

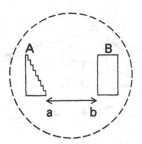

Fig. 14.27 Javal-Schiøtz keratometer. The mires.

on which the mires are mounted can be rotated about the axis of the telescope so that readings can be made in any meridian.

Doubling of the image formed by reflection at the cornea is achieved by a Wollaston prism which is incorporated in the viewing telescope. A Wollaston prism consists of two rectangular quartz prisms cemented together. Quartz is a doubly refracting substance, that is, it splits a single beam of incident light to form two polarised emergent beams. By cementing two quartz prisms together with the optical 'grain' of the crystal at right angles, it is possible to separate the two emergent beams by a fixed angle, while the dispersion produced by the first prism is neutralised by that of the second prism allowing sharp images to be formed (Fig. 14.28).

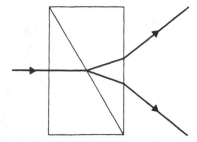

Fig. 14.28 Wollaston prism.

In order to measure corneal curvature the distance between the mires is adjusted until the doubled images just touch (fig. 14.29).

The instrument is calibrated in terms of corneal radius of curvature and in terms of dioptric refracting power of the cornea. The mires are designed so that each step of mire A

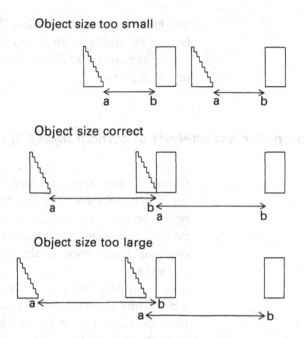

Object size too small

Object size correct

Object size too large

Fig. 14.29 Javal–Schiøtz keratometer. Appearance of images of mires.

(Fig. 14.27) is equivalent to one dioptre of corneal power. Thus if the inner images of a and b (Fig. 14.29) are aligned correctly in one corneal meridian but overlap by one and a half steps in the meridian at 90° to the first, 1.5 D of corneal astigmatism is present (Fig. 14.30a).

When an astigmatic cornea is examined, the two images are displaced vertically in all but the two principal meridians of the cornea. Thus the axis of astigmatism as well as its magnitude can be measured (Fig. 14.30b). The mires of

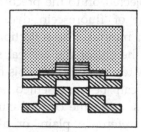

a 1½ dioptre corneal astigmatism

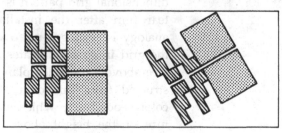

b Adjustments for reading the axis of astigmatism and corneal radius

Fig. 14.30 Javal–Schiøtz keratometer. (Haag–Streit mires) (only central pair of mires shown).

the Haag–Streit Javal–Schiøtz keratometer incorporate a horizontal line to facilitate vertical alignment.

Keratometers may also be used to measure the curvature of contact lenses.

Computerised analysis of corneal topography

Corneal topography (surface shape) can be studied by computerised analysis of the image reflected from the corneal surface. The image is analysed at thousands of points, and even minor variations in curvature can be detected. Information is obtained from a large area of the corneal surface, unlike in keratometry which obtains readings from only the central zone. The analysis of corneal topography is useful in the measurement of corneal astigmatism, contact lens fitting, refractive surgery and the early diagnosis and monitoring of keratoconus. Many patterns of corneal astigmatism are immediately apparent from a computerised image which are not revealed by refraction or keratometry.

The most common clinical method is *computerised videokeratography* (CVK). A Placido's disc is projected on to a 5- or 6 mm-diameter area of the cornea and the reflection is converted into a digital image. Where the cornea is steeper, the reflected rings lie closer together. Computer analysis produces a colour-coded contour map of the corneal surface in which locations that have the same dioptric power are indicated by the same colour.

Raster photogrammetry is a technique in which a two-dimensional grid pattern is projected on to the precorneal tear film after the installation of fluorescein dye. An analogy is casting a net over a mound. The reflection of the grid in space indicates the height of the corneal surface above a reference plane. A topographic curve is constructed from this data and can be represented as a colour-coded map which shows either the corneal curvature or the height above the reference plain, or alternatively as a three-dimensional net-like image which can be rotated in space. The image can cover all the cornea and extend on to the sclera, even if the surface is irregular or reflects poorly.

Compound microscope

A microscope provides a magnified view of a near object, as opposed to a telescope which magnifies distant objects. The compound microscope is used in many ophthalmic instruments to provide a magnified view of the eye. The slit-lamp microscope and operating microscope are obvious examples, but the keratometer and all the instruments used in conjunction with the slit-lamp, the pachometer, applanation tonometer, gonioscopy lens, etc., depend on the microscope to provide the observer with a magnified image. The specular microscope is simply a specially modified microscope which allows examination and photography of the corneal endothelium.

The compound microscope consists of two convex lenses, the objective and eyepiece lenses (Fig. 14.31). The object O to be studied is placed just outside the anterior focal point, F_o, of the objective lens OL. A real, inverted, magnified image, i, is formed some distance behind the objective lens. The eyepiece lens, EL, is placed so that the image formed by the objective falls at or close to its principal focal plane, F_e. The eyepiece thus acts as a loupe (see p. 62) and further magnifies the image seen by the observer. The final image I is vertically and horizontally inverted. Porro prisms (p. 53) are incorporated in clinical microscopes to obtain an erect noninverted image and to shorten the physical length of the instrument.

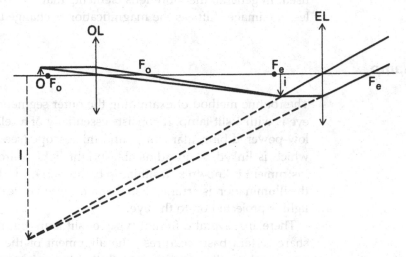

Fig. 14.31 The compound microscope.

The operating microscope and most binocular slit-lamps consist of two such compound microscopes mounted at an angle of 13° or 14° to each other, thus giving the observer a binocular, stereoscopic view. Also multiple lens elements are used, rather than two simple lenses, to reduce spherical, coma and chromatic aberration and also to achieve a smooth increase or decrease in magnification, known as zoom magnification.

The requirements of a *zoom lens system* for the operating microscope are a smooth change in magnification without changing the position of the object or image. Consider the magnification produced by a single convex lens (Chapter 5) which depends upon the distance of the object from the lens. To vary the magnification the object must be moved, and the object–image distance, or system length, also changes enormously. If the object–lens distance is to remain constant, the only way to vary the magnification is to vary the power of the lens.

In the case of the compound microscope this can be done by incorporating extra lenses which can be moved within the system, thus changing the overall power. The simplest zoom effect can be obtained by placing a single movable concave lens between the microscope lenses (Fig. 14.32) but there is significant change in image position and such a system is termed *uncompensated*.

To achieve a constant object–image distance or *compensated* zoom system, several mobile lens elements must be used. In general, the more lens elements that are used, the less the image shifts as the magnification is changed.

Slit lamp

The routine method of examining the outer segment of the eye is with a slit lamp. It consists essentially of a relatively low-powered binocular compound microscope (see above) which is linked to an adjustable bright light source. The instrument is known as a slit lamp because in everyday use the illumination is arranged so that a narrow vertical slit of light is projected on to the eye.

There are several different types of slit lamp but they all share certain basic features. The alignment of the microscope and the illumination is such that the point on which

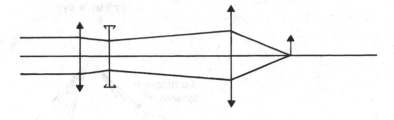

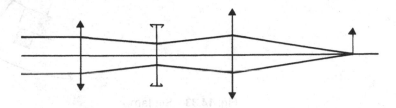

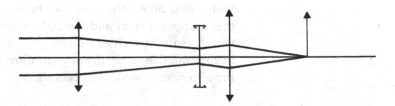

Fig. 14.32 Simple uncompensated zoom lens system.

the microscope is focused corresponds to the point on which the light is focused. This is achieved by the microscope and the lighting system having a common focal plane. Their common axis of rotation also lies in this focal plane (Fig. 14.33).

Another common feature is that there is a considerable distance between the microscope itself and the patient's eye. This is because the microscopes have a long working distance. The resulting gap between the microscope and the patient allows the observer to carry out certain manoeuvres such as removing a foreign body from the cornea. It also gives room to interpose certain optical devices, for example, a +90 D lens or a three-mirror contact lens, which permit

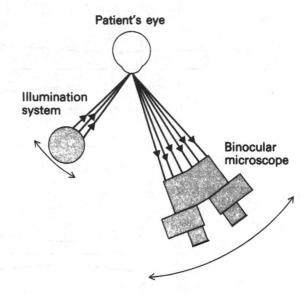

Patient's eye

Illumination system

Binocular microscope

Fig. 14.33   Slit lamp.

inspection of the vitreous and retina. The microscope tubes themselves are shortened by the incorporation of prisms, which also invert the image vertically and horizontally so that it appears erect and the right way round to the observer. A bank of Galilean telescopes of different powers is incorporated in most slit lamps to allow the magnification of the observation system to be varied.

Methods of examination

A wealth of information can be gained by examining the eye properly with a slit lamp. Certain modifications in terms of the illumination, including the use of filters, can be of considerable benefit in eliciting important physical signs.

Direct focal illumination   This is the most generally useful method of illuminating the eye. The slit beam is accurately focused upon that part of the eye under inspection.

Diffuse illumination   The beam of light is thrown slightly out of focus across the structure being examined so that a large area is diffusely illuminated. This can be a particularly helpful way of looking at the anterior capsule of the lens.

Lateral illumination This technique involves illuminating the structure being examined by light which is reflected from tissue just to one side of it. For instance, if a beam of medium width is directed upon the margin of the pupil, the outer rim of the sphincter muscle becomes apparent.

Retro-illumination This is a method of examining a particular part of the eye by light reflected from a structure behind it. The structure behind is used as a mirror to illuminate the part of the eye in question. A good example of retro-illumination is when areas of iris atrophy are identified by light which is reflected from the choroid. The illuminating column of the slit lamp should be brought to lie between the objective lenses of the microscope so that the illuminating and viewing systems are co-axial.

Specular reflection A great deal of information can be gained about the nature of a mirror-like surface by examining the rays of light reflected from it. The corneal surfaces and the anterior lens capsule can be examined in this way. Bearing in mind the laws of reflection (Chapter 2) the patient's gaze is directed to bisect the angle between the axis of illumination and that of the microscope. This is the best way of inspecting the corneal endothelium with the slit lamp.

Sclerotic scatter When the slit beam is directed on to the limbus at, for example, the 9 o'clock position, the whole limbal area glows. The maximum glow will be at the 3 o'clock position. The light from the slit beam is reflected backwards and forwards between the two internal limiting surfaces of the cornea and it is scattered centrifugally all around the cornea.

Filters

The illumination system of many slit lamps incorporates various filters. The blue cobalt filter is used during applanation tonometry (see below) and so is commonly employed.

Both the blue and the green (red-free) filters are useful in examination of the vitreous. The visibility of the gel structure of the vitreous depends upon incident light being scattered. The scattering of light is greatest when the incident light is of short wavelength. Hence blue and green light is scattered more than red light, which is of a longer wavelength.

Another reason for putting up either a blue or a green filter when inspecting the vitreous is that under these circumstances there is a relatively dark fundus background. This dark background makes it much easier to detect structures within the vitreous such as the vitreous cortex in posterior vitreous detachment. The reduced background illumination is due to only relatively few rays of shorter wavelengths being reflected from the choroid.

Fundus examination

With the basic slit lamp it is not possible to see further back into the eye than the anterior third of the vitreous. This is because the refractive power of the cornea and lens renders light emerging from the deeper points of the eye parallel. Therefore no image is formed within the focal range of the slit lamp microscope (Fig. 14.36a). However, the fundus can be rendered visible by using an additional lens to overcome the refractive power of the eye.

The view of the fundus obtained with such a lens is much improved if light reflected from the cornea does not enter the viewing system of the slit lamp microscope. This can largely be achieved if there is no overlap at the cornea of the illuminating and viewing systems.

The illumination column of most slit lamps can be tilted so that the axis of the illuminating system can be thrown below that of the viewing system (Figs. 14.34, 14.35).

Hruby lens

The Hruby lens is used to examine the fundus and posterior vitreous with the slit lamp microscope. The lens itself is a powerful plano-concave lens, −58.6 D, and it is held immediately in front of the eye under examination.

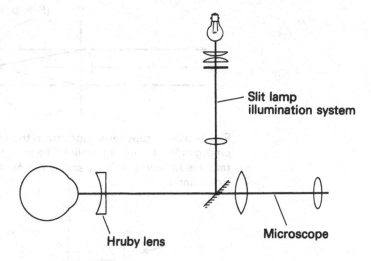

Fig. 14.34 Slit lamp. Hruby lens with coaxial illumination.

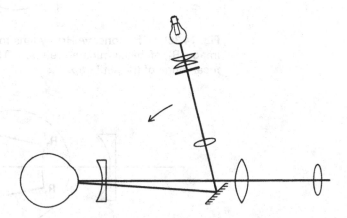

Fig. 14.35 Slit lamp. To show tilt of illumination system.

The Hruby lens works by forming a virtual, erect and diminished image of the illuminated retina, the image being anterior to the retina and within the focal range of the slit lamp microscope (Fig. 14.36).

It requires skill to use the lens. The lens is placed with its concave surface towards the eye. The best view is obtained with the lens held near the eye, when the retinal image is found in the pupillary plane.

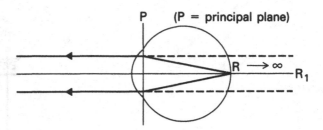

Fig. 14.36a   Hruby lens. Light from the illuminated retina, R, emerges from the eye parallel. The image R_1 of the illuminated retina is formed at infinity and is not accessible to slit lamp examination.

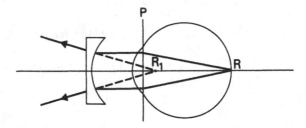

Fig. 14.36b   The concave Hruby lens forms a virtual, erect image, R_1, of the illuminated retina, R. The image lies within the focal range of the slit lamp.

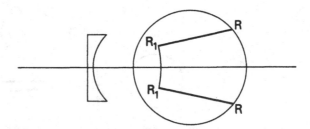

Fig. 14.36c   The virtual, erect image R_1 formed by the Hruby lens is also diminished in size, allowing a wide area of retina to be examined without undue rotation of the eye.

Fundus viewing contact lens

The fundus viewing contact lens is a device used to allow examination of the posterior vitreous and posterior pole of the fundus with the slit lamp microscope. The lens in common use is that designed by Goldmann.

The lens is a plano-concave contact lens made of material

with a higher refractive index than the eye. When applied to the cornea it allows examination of the fundus by the same mechanism as the Hruby lens.

The central zone of both the gonioscopy lens and the three-mirror contact lens (see p. 40) may also be used as a fundus viewing lens.

A plano-concave contact lens is used during vitrectomy to allow visualisation of the fundus through the operating microscope.

90 D and 78 D lenses

The principle of the indirect ophthalmoscope has been adapted so that the real image of the retina formed by the condensing lens (Fig. 14.10) may be viewed through a slit lamp microscope (Fig. 14.37). For this purpose high power condensing lenses are used, 90 D or 78 D (see Appendix II), in order to shorten the light path and bring the retinal image within the focal range of the slit lamp. The loss of image size through using such high power condensing lenses is more than compensated for by the magnification of the slit lamp microscope. The 90 D lens gives a wider field of view but less magnification than the 78 D lens. The technique gives an excellent view of the posterior pole of the fundus but is less suitable for examining the peripheral retina.

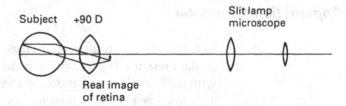

Fig. 14.37 90 D (or 78 D) lens.

Panfunduscope contact lens

A wider field of view is given by the panfunduscope contact lens (Fig. 14.38). This consists of a high convex power contact lens, which acts as a condensing lens and forms a real, inverted image of the fundus located within a spherical glass element incorporated within the panfunduscope. The spherical glass element flattens the image and redirects the

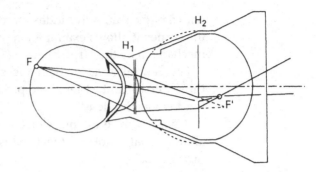

Fig. 14.38   Rodenstock panfunduscope.

light diverging from it towards the observer. Because the condensing lens is so close to the eye, the field of view is very wide. Indeed the whole fundus as far forward as the equator may be seen in one view without moving the lens. (However, the image formed is correspondingly smaller, and therefore the slit lamp must be adjusted to give high magnification if detailed examination is required.)

Other manufacturers are producing panfunduscope contact lenses which are based on the same principle as the Rodenstock lens, namely that the condensing lens is applied to the eye as a contact lens and the transmitted light collected and redirected towards the observer. The detail of the lens elements varies between manufacturers.

Applanation tonometer

The applanation tonometer is used to measure the intraocular pressure. The tonometer head is applied to the cornea with sufficient force to produce a standard area of contact. The force required is directly proportional to the intraocular pressure when the area of contact is approximately 3 mm in diameter. (When the area of contact is about 3 mm in diameter, it can be shown that the effect of surface tension (S) and the rigidity (R) of the cornea cancel each other out (Fig. 14.39). With larger areas of contact the effect of corneal rigidity becomes appreciable and leads to inaccuracy while with smaller areas of contact the surface tension causes errors.)

When the area of contact is 3.06 mm in diameter, R = S and W is proportional to P, where W is the force of application of

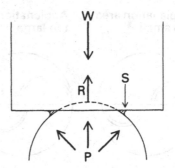

Fig. 14.39 Principle of applanation tonometry.

the tonometer; P is the intra-ocular pressure; S is the surface
tension of the tear/fluorescein ring; and R is the rigidity of
the cornea.

Furthermore, when the area of contact is 3.06 mm in
diameter, the ocular volume change caused by the tonometer is very small and does not significantly alter the intraocular pressure. A true reading of intra-ocular pressure can
thus be made.

The Goldmann and Schmidt applanation tonometer ful-
fils these conditions, the area of contact being 3.06 mm in
diameter. The instrument consists of the applanation head
which is mounted on a spring-loaded lever. The tension on
the spring is adjustable and the adjustment knob is calibrated in terms of intra-ocular pressure, in mm of mercury.

In order to achieve a standard area of corneal contact the
applanation head contains two prisms, mounted with their
bases in opposite directions (Fig. 14.40). The operator thus
looks through the applanation head and sees the circle of
corneal contact split into two half circles which are laterally
displaced in opposite directions by the prisms (Fig. 14.41).
The operator adjusts the applanation pressure until the half

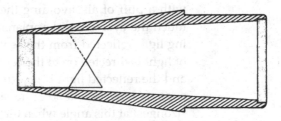

Fig. 14.40 Goldmann and Schmidt's applanation tonometer.
(Insert shows alignment of prisms.)

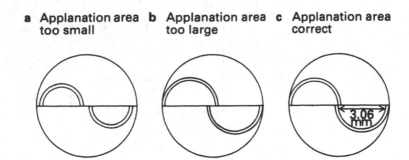

a Applanation area   **b** Applanation area   **c** Applanation area
too small   too large   correct

Fig. 14.41   Goldmann and Schmidt's applanation tonometer. Image seen by operator.

circles just overlap one another when the area of contact will be exactly 3.06 mm in diameter. (The inner edges of the fluid meniscus define the area of contact and are aligned as shown.)

If there is a high degree of corneal astigmatism, the area of contact will be elliptical, not circular, and an error of the order of 1 mmHg. per 4 dioptres of astigmatism will result. The correct area of contact will be achieved if the measurement is made at 43° to the meridian of lower corneal power (43° to the axis of the minus cylinder).

The Goldmann and Schmidt applanation tonometer has two lines marked on the tonometer prism mount, one white line in the horizontal meridian for general use, and a red line at 43° to the horizontal. The prism is marked in degrees. If the prism is mounted with the value of the axis of the minus cylinder at the red line, it is then correctly aligned to take the reading at 43° to the meridian of lower corneal power.

Non-contact tonometer

Tonometers have been developed which flatten the cornea with a puff of air, avoiding the need for the instrument to touch the eye. Corneal applanation is measured by collecting light reflected from the central cornea. A parallel beam of light is directed on to the central cornea at an angle of 30° and the reflected light is measured by a photodetector at an angle of reflection of 30°. The reflected beam of light will be strongest at this angle when the cornea is flat and acting as a plane mirror, rather than as a curved mirror. The instrument records the force of air required to flatten the cornea and displays the intraocular pressure which corresponds to that force.

The air tonometer must be used at a set distance from the cornea, and the instrument incorporates an optical alignment system to facilitate this.

Pachymeter (pachometer)

Pachymetry is the measurement of corneal thickness. Pachymeters employ either optical or ultrasound principles.

Optical pachymeters use the Purkinje–Sanson images formed by the anterior and posterior surfaces of the cornea (images I and II) to measure corneal thickness, and the Purkinje–Sanson images formed by the posterior surface of the cornea and the anterior surface of the lens (images II and III) to measure the depth of the anterior chamber. The pachymeter is attached to the slit lamp and doubles the observer's image of the field of view. Image doubling is achieved either by splitting the incident beam of light (Maurice and Giardine, Fig. 14.42) or by splitting the observer's view (Jaeger, Fig. 14.43).

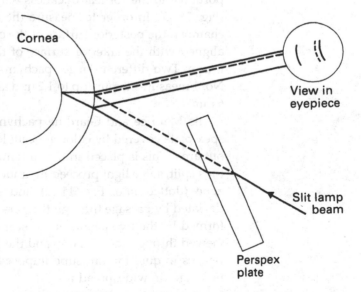

Fig. 14.42 Pachymeter of Maurice and Giardine. Measurement of corneal thickness.

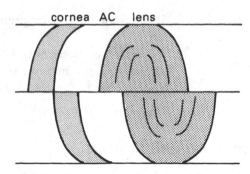

Fig. 14.43 Haag Streit (Jaeger) pachymeter. Operator's view of eye for measurement of corneal thickness.

The Jaeger pachymeter is widely used. The axis of illumination is set perpendicular to the cornea and the axis of observation is set 40° to one side of this. The observer's image of the cornea is split horizontally because it is seen through two glass plates. The lower plate is fixed but the upper one may be tilted horizontally to displace the upper half of the image (cf. oblique passage of light through a glass plate, pp. 34, 35). The observer aligns the anterior surface of the cornea in one image with its posterior surface in the second image; the degree of tilt required to do this is proportional to the corneal thickness which is read off a scale (Fig. 14.43). In order to measure the depth of the anterior chamber, the posterior surface of the cornea of one image is aligned with the anterior surface of the lens of the second image. Two different Jaeger pachymeter devices are used: No. 1 measures depths up to 1.2 mm and No. 2 depths up to 6 mm.

The Maurice and Giardine pachymeter employs a perspex plate covered by coloured celluloid and having a cutout area. This is placed in the slit lamp beam. The beam is thus split, some light proceeding undeviated via the cut-out zone (dotted line, Fig. 14.42) and some being laterally deviated by passage through the perspex plate. The images formed by the two beams at the surfaces of the cornea are viewed through the slit lamp and the plate rotated until the images in question are superimposed. This pachymeter is no longer in widespread use.

Ultrasound pachymetry allows much more precise

measurement of the corneal thickness. An ultrasound probe applanates the cornea and only gives a reading when it is perpendicular to the posterior surface. It is invaluable for planning the depth of corneal incisions in graft and refractive surgery.

Specular microscopy

Specular reflection is the reflection of light at different angles by structures with different refractive indices; the effect is more pronounced for larger differences. The angle between the axes of illumination and observation is critical and the specular reflection is therefore only viewed with one eye.

This principle is used to demonstrate any irregularity of a smooth reflecting surface occurring at the boundary of structures that have different refractive indices. For example, when the cell body and the intercellular material of the corneal endothelium are seen by specular microscopy, one appears dark, the other light. Reflection from the surface of the cornea is reduced by direct contact between the instrument and the cornea. The effect is seen by focusing on the area of interest and then carefully changing the angle of illumination. This technique is used to assess the health of a donor cornea. In the same way, lens epithelium and zones of discontinuity within the lens can be made visible.

Optical coherence tomography (OCT)

This is an experimental imaging technique analogous to B-scan ultrasound which uses the time delay of infrared light reflected by the retina to provide cross-sectional images of the retina with resolution as small as 10 μm. Light from an infrared source (843 nm) is split into a reference beam which is reflected off a mirror and a sample beam which is reflected off the retina. Temporal differences between the two reflections result in an interference signal which is processed to produce a digital image (cf. confocal scanning laser ophthalmoscope, p. 226).

Automated clinical refraction

Over the last 200 years or so attempts have been made to automate the process of refraction, but with little success. No reliable substitute could be found for the skilled human refractionist. Recently, a new generation of autorefractors has appeared on the market and it is therefore important to understand the underlying principles on which they function as well as the difficulties which prevented the successful automation of refraction in the past.

Basic principles used in automated refraction

The Scheiner principle

Scheiner discovered in 1619 that the point at which an eye was focused could be precisely determined by placing double pinhole apertures before the pupil of the eye. Parallel rays of light from a distant object are reduced to two small bundles of light by the Scheiner disc (Fig. 14.44). These form a single focus on the retina if the eye is emmetropic (Fig. 14.44a) but if there is any refractive error two spots of light fall on the retina (Figs 14.44 b–c). By adjusting the position of the object (mechanically or optically) until one focus of light is seen by the patient, the far point of the patient's eye and the refractive error can be determined. It is generally considered that the judgement of singleness of image gives a more precise endpoint than the judgement of least blur of an image.

By this method the eye is examined only along the paths of the two bundles of light transmitted by the Scheiner disc. This is the earliest of a class of 'zonal focus' methods of refraction in which the overall refractive condition is determined by examining through small zones of the optical aperture. The zonal focus methods based on the Scheiner principle have been widely used in the design of automated refractors.

The optometer principle

The term 'optometer' was first used in 1759 by Porterfield who described an instrument for 'measuring the limits of

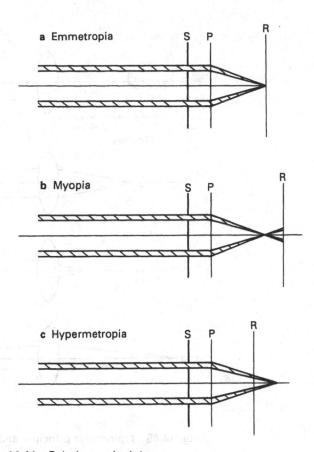

a Emmetropia   S P   R

b Myopia   S P   R

c Hypermetropia   S P   R

Fig. 14.44 Scheiner principle.

distinct vision, and determining with great exactness the strength and weakness of sight'. The principle of the optometer is illustrated in Fig. 14.45.

A convex lens is placed in front of the eye so that its focus lies in the spectacle plane and a movable target is viewed through the lens (Fig. 14.45a). If the target lies at the first principal focus of the lens, light from the target will be parallel at the spectacle plane, and focused on the retina of the emmetropic eye (Fig. 14.45b). When the target is within the focal length of the lens, light from it will be divergent in the spectacle plane (simulating a concave trial lens) (Fig. 14.45c) while light from a target outside the focal length of the lens will be convergent in the spectacle plane (simulating a convex trial lens) (Fig. 14.45d). The vergence of the light in the plane of the second principal focus of the lens is linearly related to the distance of the target from the first

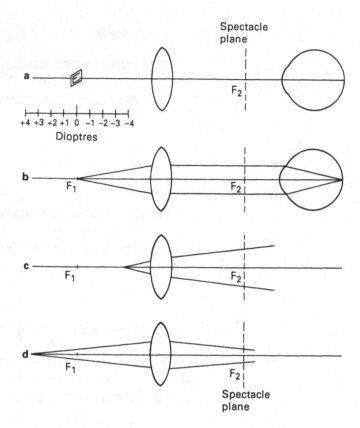

Fig. 14.45 Optometer principle and optometer.

principal focus of the lens. The instrument is calibrated to show the vergence of the light in the focal plane, in dioptres, according to the position of the target (Fig. 14.45a).

Meridional refractometry

In the presence of astigmatism, the axes of the principal meridians must be found and the refraction in both measured. This can be done even with the early instruments as long as the examiner plays an active part in the process. However, the need to identify the principal meridians of astigmatism stood in the way of truly automated refraction until the principle of meridional refractometry was discovered in the 1960s.

It was realised that if the spherical refraction is measured in at least three arbitrary meridians, the position of the principal axes and their refractive power can be found by mathematical calculation. Greater accuracy can be achieved if measurements are taken in more than three arbitrary meridians, although the mathematics becomes more complicated.

Early optometers

The earliest instruments were the subjective optometers. The patient had to adjust the instrument to achieve the best subjective focus or alignment of a target. However, the subjective optometers proved unsatisfactory because of alignment problems, irregular astigmatism and instrument accommodation.

Alignment is critical in a system based on the Scheiner principle, as both pinhole apertures must fall within the patient's pupil. Achieving and maintaining correct alignment of the instrument requires great skill and patience from the examiner and good cooperation from the patient.

Instruments using the Scheiner principle measure only the refraction of two small portions of the pupillary aperture corresponding to the apertures in the Scheiner disc. Irregular astigmatism is present to some degree in all eyes, but if it is present to a significant extent the overall refraction of the eye may be very different from the result obtained by this method.

Inappropriate accommodation often occurs when a target is viewed which is known to be within an instrument, and therefore near the eye. This is called instrument accommodation, and it has been a major problem in optometer design. Many ingenious devices have been employed in an attempt to overcome the tendency of the patient to involuntarily accommodate, but it remains a problem even in some of the modern instruments. The degree of instrument accommodation often fluctuates during the measurement process, introducing error in the astigmatic as well as the spherical correction found if the meridians are not measured simultaneously.

Between the two world wars several so-called objective optometers were developed, but these required the examiner to focus or align the image of a target on the patient's retina, so were not truly objective. They failed to come into general use because of alignment difficulties and instrument accommodation, but three of these instruments are still available and have gained acceptance in Europe where they are used in place of retinoscopy.

Infrared optometers

In recent years, the automatic infrared optometers have come to the fore. These are truly objective instruments as the instrument itself senses the end-point of refraction. Their development has sprung from the advances in electronics and microcomputers that have taken place in recent decades, and has been facilitated by the discovery of the principle of meridional refractometry.

The instruments commercially available filter out all but infrared light from the measuring system and detect the end-point by means of an electronic focus detector. Some are based on the Scheiner principle, some simulate retinoscopy and others use the optometer principle.

The patient's eye is refracted using invisible infrared light to overcome instrument accommodation. (A separate fixation target must still be provided, and is designed to encourage relaxation of accommodation.) However, because of the chromatic aberration of the eye and because infrared light is not reflected by the same layers of the retina as visible light, the refraction of the eye to infrared differs significantly from its refraction to visible light. This difference is of the order of 0.75 D to 1.50 D more hypermetropic to infrared, and may vary slightly from one individual to another. Manufacturers therefore calibrate the instruments empirically to correlate with subjective clinical results.

Furthermore, the instruments do not perform well if the eye has a small pupil or a distorted pupil, e.g. broad iridectomy, or if the ocular media are not clear (as a guideline, they become inaccurate if media haze exceeds that which would reduce the vision to 6/18).

Photoscreening

Photoscreening is a technique whereby ancillary staff, e.g. nurses or health visitors, may screen preverbal children to detect factors which may cause amblyopia. A polaroid camera in which the flash and lens are offset is used to photograph the child from a set distance in both the horizontal and vertical meridians. The alteration of the red reflex which occurs in the presence of refractive error (hypermetropia, myopia, astigmatism or anisometropia), strabismus or media opacity is captured on film. The images are examined by trained personnel, e.g. orthoptists, and can be used to select those children who should be referred to the ophthalmologist for further examination and cycloplegic refraction.

At the end of the day there is so far no machine that can equal the experienced refractionist in accuracy, ability to test abnormal eyes, patience with the very young and elderly, and wisdom to prescribe the correction that will be most suitable and acceptable to the patient.

15   Lasers

LASER is an acronym for the instrument's mode of action: Light Amplification by the Stimulated Emission of Radiation. Laser light is coherent: all photons have the same wavelength and are in phase. A laser beam is also collimated, i.e. the waves of light are parallel.

Production of laser energy

All atoms are most stable in their lowest energy state, known as the ground state (Fig. 15.1). Energy is delivered to atoms in a laser active medium by a process called pump-

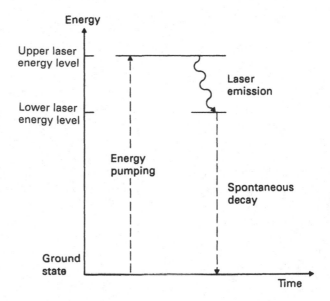

Fig. 15.1 Energy levels of a simple laser.

ing. The absorption of energy by an atom elevates its electrons from their ground state to a higher energy level. One of these, the upper laser energy level, allows excited atoms to accumulate there. When there are more atoms in the excited than in the lower energy level, population inversion is said to have occurred. Atoms in the excited state are unstable and their electrons tend to spontaneously return to the ground state by emitting light energy. This spontaneous emission of light is incoherent and it travels in all directions. Atoms are less stable in the lower laser energy state, and can drop back to the ground state and enter the cycle anew.

If an atom at a higher energy level is stimulated further by a photon whose wavelength is that which the atom would naturally emit, the resulting emission will be coherent with the stimulating photon, and the atom will drop to a lower energy level. Most of the energy released by the active medium is incoherent spontaneous emission, but the small amount released by stimulated emission can be amplified.

The active laser medium is housed in a tube which has a mirror at each end (Fig. 15.2). The distance between the mirrors must equal a multiple of the wavelengths of the light emitted so that resonance can occur. When a photon encounters an excited electron and stimulated emission occurs, the light emitted travels down the tube, and is reflected and rereflected at both mirrors. Because the mirrors are precisely aligned and a whole number of wavelengths apart, the light which has traversed the tube is still exactly in phase with itself on its second and subsequent journeys. Thus it reinforces itself. This is known as *resonance*. Meanwhile other stimulated emissions are taking place so

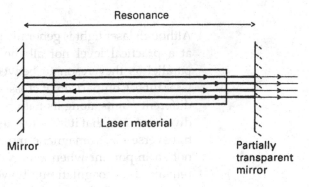

Resonance

Laser material

Mirror

Partially transparent mirror

Fig. 15.2 Laser tube.

that the light traversing the tube gets stronger and stronger while remaining exactly in phase (coherent) and the lasing process is under way.

If one of the mirrors is made partially transparent, some of the light may be allowed to leave the tube. This light will be coherent (the wavefronts in phase), monochromatic (of one wavelength) and collimated (all the rays parallel). Light is produced continuously, and such a laser is said to be operating in *continuous-wave (CW) mode*.

The actual luminous flux emitted by a laser is relatively small (lasers are very inefficient in that a great deal of energy has to be 'pumped' into them in order to maintain the lasing process). However, because the luminous flux is not scattered in all directions but is concentrated in a fine parallel beam, the beam of light is exceedingly bright. A laser producing approximately 5 lumens of light may have a beam of luminous intensity 500 million candela. Another useful comparison is that a 1 watt laser produces a retinal irradiance 100 million times greater than that of a 100 watt incandescent bulb.

Lasers are named after their active medium. The active medium contains the atoms or molecules which will undergo stimulated emission. It may be gas (argon, krypton, carbon dioxide), liquid (dye) or solid (neodymium supported by a yttrium aluminium garnet crystal, Nd:YAG). The source of the energy pumped into the active medium may be electrical discharge, a second laser or incoherent light.

Laser modes

Although laser light is generally regarded as being coherent, at a practical level not all the light waves are precisely parallel as they resonate between the two mirrors of the laser tube. Comparison of cross-sections of the laser beam at different points along its path reveals that it is very slightly divergent, and that it is more intense at certain points (called transverse electromagnetic modes). Transverse modes are not so important when energy is delivered diffusely (e.g. retinal photocoagulation); however, for photodisruption (e.g. YAG capsulotomy), it is important to have precisely focused energy to achieve a greater disruptive effect and, consequently, the effects of transverse modes need to be considered.

The point along the path of the laser beam where it is least divergent is the point at which energy can be focused to the smallest spot; this is called the fundamental mode. At the point of focus, energy is most concentrated at the centre of the laser beam and diminishes peripherally in a distribution described by a Gaussian curve (Fig. 15.3). Newer YAG laser designs increase the distribution of energy towards the centre of the beam to create a smaller point of focus and produce the same effect whilst delivering less energy.

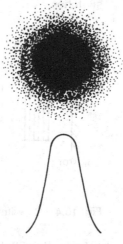

Fig. 15.3 Gaussian distribution of laser energy.

Non-fundamental modes representing divergent waves may be cancelled by an aperture inside the laser cavity to allow only the passage of parallel rays.

Mode locking, Q-switching

Power may be increased by delivering the same energy over a shorter time (power is energy per unit time, i.e. watt = joule/second). In lasers this is achieved either by mode locking or Q-switching to produce a brief pulse rather than a continuous wave of laser. The beam from a continuous wave ophthalmic laser (e.g. argon) has a constant power output and its energy output depends on the shutter speed used. Output is therefore more conveniently measured in watts. By contrast, the beam from a pulsed laser (e.g. Nd:YAG) has a peak of power and the output is therefore more conveniently measured in joules.

Q-switching is a mechanism whereby a shutter is placed in front of one of the two mirrors in the laser tube between which the oscillation of the beam normally occurs (Fig. 15.4). This maximises the energy state of the laser medium by limiting energy loss to spontaneous emission alone. Opening the shutter allows oscillation to occur and produce a single pulsed surge of stimulated emission with a duration of 2–30 nanoseconds (30×10^{-9} s). Various shutters are used, including rotating mirrors, dyes and electro-optic switches.

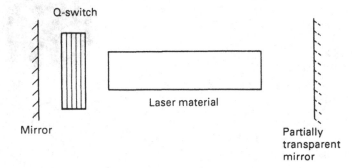

Fig. 15.4   Q-switched or mode-locked laser.

Laser light is in fact less than pure because, for several reasons, it comprises more than a single wavelength. First, the length of the laser tube, often of the order of 1 m, is enormous compared with the wavelength of laser light. It is therefore possible for multiples of several different wavelengths to 'fit' into the tube length. Secondly, in the case of solid state lasers, the heat generated during operation may cause expansion of the laser crystal, altering the distance between the mirrors. Thirdly, gas lasers have wavelength impurities caused by the Doppler effect: gas molecules have random motion and the wavelength of light which they emit depends on whether or not the direction of their random motion is the same as the emission. For these reasons, the various 'sub-wavelengths' are not in phase, a situation called free running mode. Mode locking is a refinement of Q-switching which synchronises the various wavelengths so that periodically they are in phase and summate as a train of very high energy pulses (Fig. 15.5). A pulse lasts about 30 picoseconds (30×10^{-12}s) and produces up to 100 times as much power for the same energy compared with Q-switching.

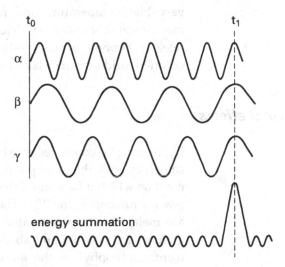

Fig. 15.5 Mode locking.

Waves α, β, γ of different wavelength normally produce destructive interference. At time intervals of t_1 they produce constructive interference and energy summation if they have already been synchronised at t_0.

Effects of laser energy on tissue

Radiation wavelengths from 400 to 1400 nm can enter the eye and reach the retina. The effects of laser energy on ocular tissues depend upon the wavelength and pulse duration of the laser light and the absorption characteristics of the tissue in question (largely determined by the pigments contained within it). When the laser energy exceeds the threshold for causing tissue damage, the mechanism for any damage depends largely upon the duration of exposure. The effects can be ionising, thermal or photochemical.

Ionisation

Photon energy delivered in a nanosecond or less may be sufficient to strip electrons from molecules to form a collection of ions and electrons called a plasma. A plasma has a very high temperature and rapidly expands to cause a mechanical shock wave sufficient to displace tissue. Energy released as photons may produce a flash. The Nd–YAG and argon–fluoride excimer lasers work in this way.

Thermal effects

Light energy is converted into heat energy if the wavelength coincides with the absorption spectrum of the tissue pigment on which it falls and if the pulse duration is between a few microseconds and 10 s. The important ocular pigments are melanin, which is located in the retinal pigment epithelium and choroid and absorbs most of the visible spectrum; xanthophyll at the macula, which strongly absorbs blue light (green is therefore safer); and haemoglobin, which absorbs blue, green and yellow wavelengths. In the retina, heat is transferred to the adjacent layers of the retina to cause a 10–20°C rise in tissue temperature. The result is photocoagulation and a localised burn. When visible or infrared light raises the tissue temperature to 100°C, water vaporises and causes tissue disruption. Carbon dioxide (CO_2) lasers also work by this mechanism: 90% of the energy is absorbed within 200 μm of the surface to which it is applied. Vaporisation may also be produced by argon retinal photocoagulation if it is too intense.

Photochemical effects

When a pulse duration of 10 s or more is required to cause damage, the mechanism is the formation of free radical ions which are highly reactive and toxic to cells. Shorter wavelengths (blue, ultraviolet) cause damage at lower levels of irradiance and are therefore more harmful. Argon lasers for retinal photocoagulation incorporate a filter to protect the operator from the photochemical effects which might otherwise be caused by reflected light.

Lasers used in ophthalmology

Every year new lasers are developed with potential uses in ophthalmology. Those described below currently have an accepted place. Laser light can be delivered along a fibre optic cable to a slit lamp, an indirect ophthalmoscope, or an intraocular endolaser probe.

The argon blue-green gas laser

The argon blue-green gas laser emits a mixture of 70% 488 nm (blue) and 30% 514 nm (green) light. Argon lasers are most commonly employed for retinal photocoagulation. Older models were large and required a water cooling system to dissipate the heat generated. Newer lasers are smaller and air cooled, and limit emission to green light for a number of reasons. Photocoagulation aims to treat the outer retina and spare the inner retina to avoid damaging the nerve fibre layer. Argon green (blue screened out) photocoagulation of the macula does not cause direct retinal damage. Argon green is well absorbed by melanin and haemoglobin. Xanthophyll in the inner layer of the macula absorbs blue light (but not green) and thus the use of blue light at the macula is contraindicated in order to avoid direct damage to the retina in this region. Scattering of the laser light by the crystalline lens of older individuals affects the focus of the beam and necessitates the use of much higher power settings.

The He–Ne laser

The helium-neon (He–Ne) laser is a low power gas laser whose visible red 632.8 nm emission is used as an aiming beam for lasers with invisible output (e.g. Nd–YAG, diode).

Diode lasers

The diode lasers emit a wavelength of 810 nm infrared in continuous wave mode. The laser energy is generated by a semiconductor diode chip. Diode lasers are efficient, generate little excess heat and are portable. In the eye, diode laser light is absorbed only by melanin and consequently is most commonly used for retinal photocoagulation. Low scattering of this wavelength ensures good penetration of the ocular media and of oedematous retina. The 810 nm wavelength also penetrates the sclera. Thus, even if the retina is obscured from view through the pupil, photocoagulation may still be performed by placing the delivering probe on the surface of the eye. The transparency of the sclera to diode laser also allows photocycloablation of the ciliary body in 'end stage' glaucoma. Diode photocoagulation of vascular structures (e.g. neovascular membranes and tumours) is enhanced by intravenous indocyanine green dye with an absorption peak of 800–810 nm. Diode laser light has been used endoscopically to create a dacryocystorhinostomy (DCR).

The Nd–YAG laser

The neodymium–yttrium–aluminium–garnet (Nd–YAG) laser emits 1064 nm infrared radiation. It is a powerful continuous wave (CW) laser which is usually Q-switched when used to treat the eye. It is commonly used to disrupt the posterior capsule of the lens following cataract surgery, or the iris in narrow angle glaucoma. Laser energy is emitted from neodymium molecules which are suspended in a clear YAG crystal to achieve a higher concentration of Nd ions than is possible in a gas laser medium. The 1064 nm wavelength is invisible and requires a He–Ne laser red aiming beam. Before use on a patient's eye, the operator must ensure that the laser beam and the aiming beam are focused at the same point.

The frequency-doubled Nd-YAG laser

The frequency-doubled Nd-YAG laser emits 532 nm radiation. This is achieved by passing 1064 nm radiation from a YAG crystal through a potassium titinyl phosphate (KTP) crystal, thereby converting some of the energy to 532 nm radiation. The YAG crystal may be pumped by arc light or by a diode laser. The photocoagulation effect is similar to that of continuous wave argon green laser.

The excimer laser

The excimer laser derives its name from 'excited dimer', two atoms forming a molecule in the excited state but which dissociate in the ground state. Excimer lasers in clinical use employ an argon–fluorine (Ar–F) dimer laser medium to emit 193 nm ultraviolet (UV) radiation. High absorption of UV by the cornea limits its penetration. Each photon has 6.4 eV, sufficient to break intramolecular bonds. The delivery of a relatively high level of energy to a small volume of tissue causes tissue removal (i.e. ablation). The ablation depth may be precisely determined. Although the temperature in a tiny volume of treated tissue becomes very high, the amount of heat produced is very small and there is no significant rise in temperature of adjacent tissue. The excimer laser is therefore ideally suited to photorefractive keratectomy (PRK) and laser intrastromal keratomileusis (LASIK) to reshape the corneal surface (cf. Chapter 17) as well as phototherapeutic keratectomy (PTK) to remove abnormal corneal surface tissue.

The erbium:YAG laser

The erbium:YAG laser delivers 2940 nm infrared radiation which is absorbed by water and penetrates tissue by less than 1 µm. The absorption of energy by a very small volume of tissue results in the explosive evaporation of tissue, and thermal effects are limited to the surrounding 5–15 µm. This laser has been used experimentally to emulsify the lens in cataract surgery.

The carbon dioxide laser

The carbon dioxide (CO_2) laser emits 10600 nm mid-infrared wavelength which is strongly absorbed by water, and therefore by most tissues. The only effects are thermal; the diffusion of heat from the target coagulates adjacent tissues, and water vaporisation releases steam. Such lasers are used in other branches of surgery to produce a nearly bloodless incision but have yet to find a use in ophthalmology.

Investigational applications of lasers in ophthalmology

Confocal optics

When an imaging and illumination system focus on the same small point, the system is described as being confocal. The contrast and resolution of the image are increased by minimising the amount of scattered light by means of a very small area of illumination and field of view. This is achieved by using a laser source of illumination and by the observer viewing through a pinhole or slit. The overall field of view is then increased by scanning across the area being examined.

Confocal microscopy

The principle of confocal optics is used in laser scanning confocal miscroscopy, a means of looking in microscopic detail at different depths of the living cornea.

Confocal scanning laser ophthalmoscope

The confocal scanning laser ophthalmoscope (CSLO) employs confocal optics to image the optic nerve head and retina. Different laser sources have been used: Ar blue (488 nm), Ar green (514 nm), HeNe red (633 nm) and diode infrared (780 nm). The CSLO has also been used to perform fluorescein and indocyanine green angiography and microperimetry (see below).

Scanning laser polarimetry

This is a technique of measuring the thickness of the retinal nerve fibre layer (RNFL) by exploiting its birefringence. A CSLO projects a spot of polarised laser light (780 nm) on to the retina which passes through the RNFL to the deeper retinal structures, from where it is partly reflected back through the RNFL to leave the eye. The RNFL behaves as a birefringent medium because the axons are arranged in parallel and change the state of polarisation of the light passing through it. The magnitude of change of polarisation is called retardation and correlates with the thickness of the RNFL. This information is used to evaluate RNFL damage caused by glaucoma.

Confocal scanning laser tomography

This technique uses a CSLO (diode 670 nm) to produce a topographic map of the optic nerve head. Only light reflected from the surface of the retina lying in the focal plane of the scanning laser beam is imaged. Each image is formed by a grid of tiny squares called pixels. The first of the 32 images acquired is in the plane which is parallel to the surface of the retina, just anterior to the blood vessels as they emerge from the optic cup. Subsequent images are acquired by advancing the focal plane posteriorly to the lamina cribrosa. A plane is chosen as the reference plane and the height of each pixel above it is calculated. A computer converts this information into a three-dimensional reconstruction which can be used to evaluate disc damage in glaucoma.

Laser interferometry

Interferometers project laser light (usually He–Ne) from two sources on to the retina. Interference occurs where the two beams meet and is seen as a sine wave grating. This effect occurs despite the presence of a cataract or refractive error. Reducing the separation between the light sources reduces the spatial frequency of the sine wave grating and allows the estimation of the potential visual acuity of an eye when the macula cannot be seen because of a cataract.

Laser microperimetry

This technique uses a laser beam to determine the light sensitivity of very small areas of the retina and to identify small scotomas.

Laser Doppler flowmetry

This is a means of measuring retinal capillary blood flow. It is based on the Doppler principle. Laser light incident upon moving blood cells is reflected at a different frequency from the incident beam. A greater shift in frequency indicates a greater blood flow velocity.

The Holmium laser

The Holmium laser has been used to create a sclerostomy to increase aqueous humour outflow in the treatment of glaucoma and in thermokeratoplasty to change the surface curvature of the cornea.

The Nd:YLF laser

The neodymium–yttrium–lithium–fluoride (Nd:YLF) laser emits 1053 nm with a picosecond (10^{-12} s) pulse duration which can be delivered at a very high repetition rate. It can be used experimentally to dissect rather than disrupt tissue, and has been used to create sclerostomies, dissect vitreous membranes and change refractive errors by the intrastromal ablation of the cornea.

Laser safety

The eye is at far greater risk from the potentially damaging effects of optical radiation than other areas of the body because its optical properties focus the beam on the retina, increasing the irradiance by as much as 10^5. Lasers are therefore classified according to their potential to damage the eye (Table 15.1). All surgical lasers, including those used in ophthalmology, are capable of damaging the eye and are classified as 3b or 4. It is essential that their effects be limited to the therapeutic end desired, and that accidental damage is not inflicted on the patient, the surgeon or other persons in the vicinity. To this end there are strict safety regulations which must be adhered to.

Table 15.1   International safety classification of lasers.

Class	Output (mW)		Safety
1	≤0.0004 ≤0.024	*blue or green* *red*	Eye safe Eye safe
2	<1	*visible wavelengths*	Eye safe – brightness causes blink and aversion
3a	1–5	*visible wavelengths*	Eye safe – brightness causes blink and aversion
3b	5–500		Significant eye damage, e.g. retinal photocoagulation
4	≥500		Serious irreversible damage, e.g. medical, industrial, military

Where there is a risk to the surgeon from reflected laser light, protection is provided by shutters or filters built into the instrument which operate when the laser is fired. The filters absorb the laser light but transmit enough light of other wavelengths to allow the effect of the laser on the target to be observed. The laser area should be free of personnel but, if attendance of other individuals is essential, protective goggles should be used.

16   Practical Clinical Refraction

Having assimilated the optical theory presented in the previous chapters, the practitioner should be able to approach the refraction of a patient understanding the principles of what he is doing. But is this enough? Experienced refractionists know that prescribing is an art as well as a science. There are certain clinical tips that have been handed down over the years, respect for which makes the difference between the mediocre and good refractionist. Some of these will be included in the following sections on practical refraction and are printed in italics.

History

The patient's age and occupation and special visual requirements, e.g. occupation and hobbies, must be ascertained. Visual symptoms, eye-related diseases and family history of eye disease, especially glaucoma, must be enquired for. The patient's past history of spectacle wear is important, and it is wise to find out the previous prescription, if this is available, and to examine the old glasses. *Note the lens form of the previous glasses. Myopes are especially intolerant of a change in lens form and some prefer to continue wearing planoconcave lenses, known as 'flats', even though this may not be the best form of lens for their prescription. Notice the type of multifocal lenses in use and whether the patient is happy with them.*

Examination

The visual acuity is measured uniocularly for distance and near, unaided and with existing spectacles. *Fog the fellow eye of patients with nystagmus with a high plus lens as complete occlusion makes the nystagmus worse and lowers the uniocular acuity.* If the acuity is very poor, examine briefly with the ophthalmoscope at this stage to exclude a pathological cause. *More detailed scrutiny of the fundi should be left until after the refraction to avoid photostress-induced reduction of acuity.*

Objective refraction

Perform the cover/uncover test to detect any manifest squint. *If the patient has a manifest squint without diplopia, binocular vision is lacking and it will not be possible to test the muscle balance by the Maddox rod and wing tests (see below) which depend on binocular vision.*

Fit the trial frame, taking care that the lens apertures are centred on the pupils with the patient gazing straight ahead. The frame must be level across the face, and as close to the eyes as the lashes will allow. Remember always to place high power trial lenses in the back cell of the trial frame (cf. effective power of lenses and back vertex distance, p. 125).

Perform the retinoscopy with the patient gazing at a distant object, such as the top letter of the test type. It is important to perform the retinoscopy as close to the patient's visual axis as possible in order to measure the true optical length of the eye. Care should be taken to ensure that the patient's view of the distant fixation object is not obstructed. To this end the examiner should ideally use his right eye to examine the patient's right eye and his left eye for the patient's left eye. If the examiner does get in the way, the patient loses distant fixation and may start to accommodate. (*If the patient does accommodate and fix on the examiner, this will be betrayed because the pupil will constrict and the retinoscopy reflex become more difficult to see.*) During retinoscopy it is considered better to fog the patient's fellow eye rather than to occlude it in order to discourage involuntary accommodation. In the presence of manifest squint the dominant eye may have to be occluded to achieve steady fixation with the non-dominant eye.

In the case of young children, or children who have a latent or manifest squint, the ciliary muscle should be paralysed with a topical cycloplegic drug before retinoscopy is performed. This allows the true magnitude of any refractive error to be determined (see p. 114, hypermetropia).

Some refractionists place a plus lens of the dioptric value of their working distance (e.g. +1.50 DS for $\frac{2}{3}$ metre) in the trial frame before commencing the retinoscopy. Once the point of reversal or neutral point (see p. 186) has been reached for both eyes, this lens is removed and the subjective examination started with the lenses remaining in the frame.

After viewing the retinoscopy reflex through the working distance lens, further spherical lenses are added, convex if the movement is 'with' and concave if 'against' (Fig. 16.1a–c) until the neutral point is reached in one meridian (Fig. 16.1d). (If this lies between increments of lens power, reversal of the reflex movement is taken as the end point.) Cylindrical lenses may then be used to neutralise the other meridian and to find the axis of the astigmatism present.

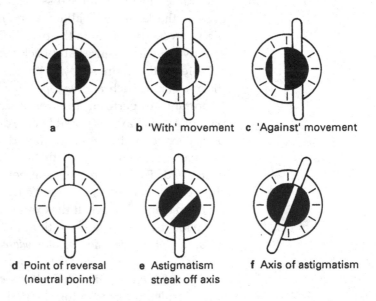

a   **b** 'With' movement   **c** 'Against' movement

d Point of reversal (neutral point)   **e** Astigmatism streak off axis   **f** Axis of astigmatism

Fig. 16.1 Retinoscopy reflexes.

The axis may be found because the retinoscopy reflex will only align with the axis of the cylindrical lens (and the retinoscopy streak if a streak retinoscope is being used) when they all lie in the axis of the astigmatism. If the axis of the cylindrical lens lies outside the axis of astigmatism, the reflex will move obliquely (Fig. 16.1e). As the point of reversal is approached, it can be shown that the angle of misalignment of the reflex will be six times the angle of misalignment of the cylindrical lens. The cylinder, therefore, must be rotated by only a small amount before rechecking the retinoscopy, and this method provides a very accurate means of determining the axes of astigmatism objectively.

The same method may also be used to identify the axes of astigmatism if spherical lenses alone are used during retinoscopy, e.g. during cycloplegic retinoscopy of a small child when it is easier to hold lenses in the hand rather than use a trial frame. The reflex in the pupil will only align with the streak when both lie in one principal meridian of astigmatism (Fig. 16.1d–e).

It is often said that minus cylinders should be used during retinoscopy because the use of plus cylinders when refracting young hypermetropic patients may stimulate accommodation as the eye is fogged in both meridians only when the full plus cylinder is in place. However, if minus cylinders are always used, there is a tendency to overcorrect hypermetropia in the elderly and when performing cycloplegic refraction. This is because most patients will not accept the full value of the cylinder found on retinoscopy. Supposing that at the end of retinoscopy, after correction for working distance, the trial frame contains a +4.00 DS and a –1.50 DC. On subjective refraction the patient tolerates only a –1.00 DC, so the frame now contains +4.00 DS and –1.00 DC. With this combination of lenses the lower value meridian is overcorrected by +0.50 D and the examiner must verify the spherical correction again, reducing it to +3.50 DS. If, however, the lenses used for the retinoscopy had been +2.50 DS and +1.50 DC, after reduction of the cylinder to +1.00 DC, the higher value meridian would be undercorrected, which is better tolerated, and the spherical correction would not need to be changed.

Some refractionists therefore prefer to use plus cylinders with plus spheres, and minus cylinders with minus spheres. Thus retinoscopy is performed with spheres up to the lowest meridian of reversal, and continued with cylinders of the same sign to the higher meridian of reversal. The exception to this is when the initial (uncorrected) retinoscopy reflexes move in opposite directions in the two meridians, i.e. one 'with' and one 'against'. In this case, spherical lenses are added until one meridian is neutralised, and cylindrical lenses of opposite sign and higher power are added until the other meridian is neutralised. *It is wise to use minus spheres and plus cylinders for this purpose because it is easier to find the axis of astigmatism using the 'with' movement seen when plus cylinders are being added than the 'against' movement that goes with the use of plus spheres and minus cylinders.*

The retinoscopy findings are usually recorded in the UK according to the following convention (Fig. 16.2).

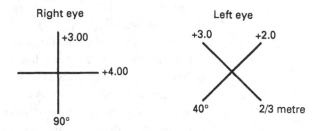

Fig. 16.2   Record of retinoscopy findings.

A cross is drawn in the orientation of the principal meridians, and the angle of one meridian marked. The dioptric value of the point of reversal is marked on each meridian and the working distance recorded. If this result is transposed into a lens prescription (corrected for working distance) the axis of any cylinder lies at 90° to the line of its meridian. For example, the left eye in Fig. 16.2 would be

$$\frac{+0.50 \text{ DS}}{+1.00 \text{ DC axis } 40°} \quad \text{or} \quad \frac{+1.50 \text{ DS}}{-1.00 \text{ DC axis } 130°}$$

In practice retinoscopy is not always easy.

In cases of high refractive error, the initial reflex may be too dim and diffuse to be identified. Retinoscopy should be repeated using a moderately strong convex and concave lens, e.g. + or –7.00 DS, one of which should bring the reflex into view, assuming that the media are clear. Alternatively, examination of the eye with the direct ophthalmoscope will allow differentiation between high myopia and high hypermetropia.

If the refraction varies between the central and peripheral

parts of the pupillary aperture, there may be an increase in brightness in the centre or periphery due to spherical aberrations. For example, in nucleosclerosis the central zone is relatively myopic compared with the periphery and the centre of the pupil appears bright. To judge the end-point, which may not be as sharply defined as usual, concentrate on the central zone in which the visual axis lies.

It is sometimes difficult to decide whether the reflex is moving 'with' or 'against' the movement of the retinoscope because there appear to be two reflexes in the pupil, moving towards and away from each other like the blades of a pair of scissors, so-called 'scissor shadows' (Fig. 16.3a). This is due to a difference in refraction between different zones of the pupillary aperture. It is more commonly seen with a dilated pupil and near the end-point of retinoscopy, when one area will be relatively myopic, M, while the other is relatively hypermetropic, H, to the plane of observation, R (Fig. 16.3b). It is traditionally taught that the end-point is taken when the two reflexes meet in the centre of the pupil, but this may be difficult to judge. In our experience, one blade of the scissors is brighter than the other and the end-point is taken when the brighter reflex reverses.

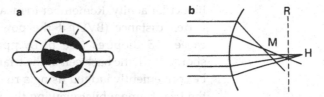

Fig. 16.3 Retinoscopy. (a) Scissor shadows. (b) Optical diagram to show cause of scissor shadows.

Retinoscopy may be very difficult in keratoconus, when a characteristic swirling reflex is seen and the reflex from the apex of the cone is darker than the periphery (the oil-drop sign). It may be impossible to detect an end-point, and subjective testing must then be relied upon.

Subjective refraction

Make the correction for your working distance (add −1.50 DS for $\frac{2}{3}$ metre or remove the 'working distance lens' if one was used) *and, because patients usually do not tolerate the full cylindrical correction, it helps to reduce the cylinder by approximately a quarter of its value (see above)* before commencing the subjective examination.

Occlude the fellow eye (unless nystagmus is present, in which case use a fogging technique, pp. 230, 231). Using the distance test type, first verify the sphere by offering small plus and minus additions until no further improvement can be made. Patients with good visual acuity can appreciate a difference of 0.25 DS while those with poor acuity may only appreciate larger increments, e.g. 0.50 DS. Next verify the axis of the cylinder before adjusting its power (cf. the cross-cylinder, Chapter 6, pp. 71–73). If a large change is found in the cylinder, it is wise to go back and recheck the sphere. If the patient is myopic, the duochrome test (Chapter 8, pp. 90–92) should be done monocularly and binocularly.

If the red letters are only marginally clearer than the green when the patient views them monocularly, the green letters may be clearer when the eyes are used together. A small reduction, e.g. +0.25 DS, to one or both eyes may be needed to make the red letters clearer binocularly and ensure that the patient will be comfortable, and not accommodating, when wearing the prescription.

Record the prescription and acuity for each eye, and the binocular acuity. Remember to measure and record the back vertex distance (BVD) if the power of the spherical lens exceeds 5 dioptres (see BVD, pp. 101, 125). Such a lens should be in the back cell of the trial frame and the BVD may be conveniently judged using a ruler held beside the arm of the trial frame whilst viewing the patient from the side.

Use the Maddox rod (Chapter 6, pp. 67–69) to check the muscle balance for distance. *Some patients are initially unable to see the white spotlight and the red line, especially if there is confusing side illumination in the room. Occlude each eye in turn to ascertain that the spot and line are visible to the appropriate eye uniocularly, and then uncover both eyes and see if the patient is able to perceive them simultaneously. If the patient sees them one at a time uniocularly but not simultaneously with both eyes uncovered, his binocular vision must be defective or absent.* In cases where the Maddox rod test reveals a significant extraocular muscle imbalance, especially a vertical one, check to see if the addition of the appropriate prism improves the patient's binocular comfort and acuity. *The full value of prism as found by the Maddox rod test is rarely required.*

If the patient is presbyopic, calculate the likely reading addition and add this to the distance lenses in the trial frame. In practice the reading addition is estimated by rule-of-thumb from the patient's age:

> 45–50 years = +1.00 D addition
> 50–55 = +1.50 D addition
> 55–60 = +2.00 D addition
> over 60 = +2.50 D addition

Beware of prescribing too great a reading addition (cf. Chapter 11). *The most frequent reason that patients seek a retest is that too strong a near addition has been prescribed. In normal circumstances not more than +2.50 DS addition should be given. However, pseudophakic patients often prefer a +3.00 DS addition.* Record the near acuity for each eye alone and binocularly.

Use the Maddox wing to check the near muscle balance. Orthophoria for distance but a large exophoria for near indicates convergence insufficiency. This may cause such symptoms as headache or eye-strain after close work, or it may be asymptomatic. If the patient has symptoms, the convergence should be strengthened by means of convergence exercises. *If base-in prisms are prescribed, the convergence may become weaker still, and progressively stronger prisms will be required.* Vertical muscle imbalances for near may require prismatic correction, but again the full value of prism is rarely required or tolerated.

Measurement of interpupillary distance

It is sometimes useful to measure the patient's interpupillary distance, although this is usually done in the UK by the dispensing optician. The measurement of the interpupillary distance is important in babies and small children, especially if high power lenses have been prescribed, as decentration caused by an unsuitable spectacle frame will introduce an unwanted prismatic effect (cf. spherical lens decentration, p. 64, and prism power, p. 43). Poor centration of aphakic spectacle lenses also causes an unwanted prismatic effect and this is a common cause of intolerance of aphakic glasses.

The anatomical interpupillary distance may be measured by the following methods. A millimetre rule is rested across the bridge of the patient's nose and the patient asked to look at the examiner's left eye. The zero of the rule is aligned with the nasal limbus of the patient's right eye (which will be looking straight ahead at the examiner's left eye). The patient is then instructed to look at the examiner's right eye and the position of the temporal limbus of the patient's left eye is noted, giving the anatomical interpupillary distance. (The measurements are taken from limbus to limbus to exclude inaccuracy due to differences or changes in pupil size.) Alternatively, a fixation light may be held in front of each of the examiner's eyes in turn and a similar procedure followed, the distance between the corneal light reflexes on the patient's eyes being measured.

The measurement of importance in making spectacles is the distance between the visual axes for distance vision which is approximately 1 mm less than the anatomical interpupillary distance.

Helpful hints to avoid intolerance

- Do not change the axis of the cylinder, especially in a myope, unless there are compelling reasons for doing so.
- Do not change the lens form worn by a myope.
- Do not prescribe a large cylinder for any patient who has never worn a cylindrical correction before. Break them in gradually. The exception to this is pseudophakic patients who tolerate a full astigmatic correction well.
- Do not overcorrect hypermetropes: better to leave them 0.25 DS undercorrected so they can read the bus numbers in the far distance.
- Do not fully correct myopes: better to leave them 0.25 DS undercorrected so they do not have to use their accommodation for distance.
- Do not give too great a reading addition, so the patient cannot read the newspaper held at arm's length (cf. p. 143).
- Do not recommend bifocal or progressive lenses without carefully considering the needs, occupation and frailties of the patient.
- Discuss with the patient the subjective and practical

points relevant to the new prescription, e.g. warn a new bifocal wearer to be careful at steps.
- Do not alter a satisfactory prescription unless there is a very definite reason to do so.
- Do not advise patients to buy new glasses because of a minor change in prescription that they will not be able to appreciate subjectively.

Notes on the management of refractive errors in children

The refraction and management of children with refractive errors is possibly the most interesting and rewarding aspect of the refractionist's work. The following discussion relates to the management of the age group at risk of developing squint or amblyopia, e.g. birth to approximately 8 years of age.

As stated above, cycloplegic refraction is necessary to obtain an accurate retinoscopy in infants and children. If this is done, some degree of ametropia will be found in most cases and judgement must be exercised to decide whether spectacles will be beneficial. (Most parents hope their children will not need glasses, and the children tolerate glasses better if they perceive that they see better when wearing them.)

Hypermetropia is very common in infants and children, and requires a full correction in the presence of esophoria or esotropia. It is also wise to correct it if there is a family history of esotropia. Moderate or high degrees of hypermetropia require correction to achieve good visual acuity, and more than 1 dioptre of hypermetropic anisometropia must be corrected to prevent refractive amblyopia in the more hypermetropic eye (cf. p. 116).

The uncorrected hypermetropic child overcomes some or all of his hypermetropia by exercising extra accommodation. When glasses are worn for the first time, the accommodation may not relax and the vision will be blurred. Usually the accommodation relaxes after a few days if the glasses are persevered with, but it is wise to warn the parents about this when the glasses are prescribed. Occasionally the accommodation fails to relax and the prescription needs to be reduced for a while, or a short course of cycloplegic drops may do the trick.

Myopia of sufficient degree to prevent the child from seeing what is written on the blackboard should be corrected before the child starts formal schooling. Myopia should also be corrected in the presence of exophoria or exotropia in order to stimulate accommodation and convergence.

It is wise to explain to the parents that the glasses will have to be made stronger as the child grows bigger, because the eye also grows, and this progression of the myopia should not be a cause of undue concern and will stabilise when growth stops.

High myopia should be corrected as soon as it is detected because it impairs the child's perception of the environment and may retard development in many fields, e.g. mobility, relating to other people, recognising shapes and objects and learning to use the hands, etc. *Experience shows that in both adults and children a full correction is not tolerated in high myopia. Such patients should be left 1 or 2 dioptres undercorrected.*

Uniocular moderate or high myopia often causes amblyopia and an attempt should be made to correct it. Surprisingly good results can be achieved with spectacles, if started early, even in high degrees of anisometropia as the young brain seems to cope with much greater degrees of aniseikonia than the adult is able to. Sometimes a contact lens for a unilateral highly myopic eye will be effective where glasses have failed, but the age and suitability of the child and family must be taken into account as contact lens wear entails practical problems, especially in children.

Astigmatism needs correction if the visual acuity is reduced in the affected eye. Most babies and many infants have quite high degrees of astigmatism but in many cases this reduces or disappears by the age of $2\frac{1}{2}$ or 3 years when the first accurate tests of visual acuity become possible. Astigmatism alone rarely needs correction in infants. In children of 3 years of age and older, astigmatism of 1 dioptre or more, which is sufficient to impair the visual acuity, should be corrected.

Remember to check the fit of the frames for sore spots or chafing if a child refuses to keep his glasses on. It is worth telling the parents to do this when new glasses are acquired as non-spectacle wearers may not think of this as a cause of non-tolerance.

Once a child is established in glasses, it is usual to review the refraction annually. If the visual acuity is good with the existing prescription and the child is cooperative, cycloplegic refraction may not be necessary. Retinoscopy performed through the existing glasses with the child fixing a distant target and fogged with +1.50 D lenses (for a working distance of $\frac{2}{3}$ metre) will show whether there is sufficient change in the spectacle prescription to necessitate a more careful refraction.

17   Refractive Surgery

The goal of surgery to correct a refractive error should be to safely and predictably create a stable and desired refractive state without causing new optical problems. Patients request refractive surgery because other methods of optical correction are inconvenient, are not tolerated, or are optically or cosmetically unsatisfactory. A few may wish to pursue a career or pastime which is not possible with their refractive error. Not all those seeking refractive surgery are suitable candidates. Other methods of optical correction may be more appropriate, the patient's expectations may be unreasonably high or there may be an ocular or systemic condition which first requires treatment or makes refractive surgery inappropriate. Patients should be made aware of the alternatives and of the complications associated with the procedure to be undertaken and also the probability of achieving the desired refractive outcome.

For most patients, the preferred outcome of refractive surgery is emmetropia whereby the far point of the eye is at infinity. Correction of myopia requires the reduction of the refractive power of the eye; for hypermetropia it must be increased. There are several ways to alter the refractive state of the eye: by changing the refractive power of any of the ocular media, the depth of the anterior chamber or the axial length of the eye. Most of the refractive power of the eye occurs at the air–cornea interface and there are numerous techniques to reshape the corneal surface. The crystalline lens is the second most important refractive element in the eye, and modern cataract surgery allows quite a predictable refractive outcome but accommodation is eliminated. Almost any spherical refractive error can be corrected by replacing the crystalline lens with an intraocular lens. Corneal surgery is usually limited to correcting refractive errors in the range +4.00 to –10.00 D. This is because of the greater likelihood of corneal scarring and the reduced predictability of outcome with larger refractive errors.

The intended refractive outcome of surgery is decided after carefully discussing the patient's visual requirements and taking account of the potential visual acuity. The refractive error of the fellow eye and whether this eye is also likely to require surgery must be considered. The timing of surgery is also important. In most instances the preferred outcome is emmetropia, but for patients who wish to dispense with glasses for near, one might aim for –2.50 D. Some surgeons aim for a refractive outcome of –1.00 D to allow an uncorrected acuity which is reasonable for both near and distance. This approach allows for a margin of error and makes it less likely that the eye will become hypermetropic, which patients greatly dislike.

The consequences of creating anisometropia must be considered in patients who have reasonably good corrected visual acuity in each eye. They are unlikely to tolerate anisometropia of more than 2.50 D unless they tolerate a contact lens in the unoperated eye. Work requiring stereopsis and good visual acuity may therefore become impossible. The alternatives are enduring anisometropia until the fellow eye is operated upon, making the first eye less ametropic and the second even less so, and lastly, monovision whereby one eye is emmetropic and used for distance and the other is myopic and used for near. As many as 50% of patients are unable to adapt to monovision. Patients with poor corrected vision in one eye can usually be made emmetropic in the other without causing intolerable anisometropia. Myopes of long standing frequently wish to be left mildly myopic if they are used to performing near tasks without optical correction, and may find emmetropia and the requirement for convex lenses for near tasks difficult to adjust to.

Many forms of surgery have the potential to affect refraction to some degree by causing one or more of these changes. A greater understanding of the effects of ocular incisions and suture placement on corneal astigmatism and topography has done much to reduce inconvenient postoperative refractive errors but the effects of scleral buckles, silicone oil and intraocular gas used in vitreoretinal surgery are often unavoidable.

The refractive error and corneal topography should be stable before considering a procedure to change the refractive state of the cornea. Childhood myopia may not stabilise until the third decade, and 21 years is therefore considered the lower acceptable age limit. PMMA hard contact lenses, gas permeable lenses and soft contact lenses have been shown to cause corneal warpage. Corneal topography changes for an average of fifteen, ten and five weeks respectively after contact lens wear is discontinued, and refractive surgery should not be undertaken before the topography has stabilised. Some patients may consider this an unacceptably long interval and refuse surgery.

Photorefractive keratectomy (PRK)

This technique uses an excimer laser (cf. p. 225) to change the anterior curvature of the cornea. Each laser pulse ablates tissue from the surface of the cornea to a depth of 0.4–0.5 microns. The diameter of the laser beam may vary between a fraction of 1 mm and 7 mm and is controlled by an aperture. A computerised algorithm controls the treatment parameters.

To correct myopia successive concentric applications of increasing diameter are made so that more tissue is ablated centrally than peripherally and the surface curvature is reduced. If the diameter of the area treated is of the order 3.5–4 mm, the edge may cause haloes to be seen around lights when the pupil is dilated. A wider area of treatment, e.g. 6–7mm, makes this less likely but requires deeper ablation to achieve the same refractive outcome. A strategy to correct higher degrees of myopia using a wide treatment area whilst minimising the depth entails multiple concentric treatment zones and smoothing the transition between them; only the centremost zone provides full dioptric correction. More highly myopic eyes have a less predictable refractive outcome, a greater likelihood of late regression towards myopia and increased risk of sub-epithelial scarring which can cause glare or reduce the best corrected visual acuity.

Alternatives to a broad excimer laser beam are a scanning slit or a flying dot, which have lower energy output but a prolonged treatment time and therefore require a system to fix or track the position of the eye.

It is more difficult to correct an astigmatic than a spherical refractive error. Regular astigmatism is corrected by reducing the surface curvature more in the steepest meridian than in any other. This can be accomplished using a slit beam, an elliptical ablation zone, a scanning beam or an ablatable mask. As a slit beam widens for successive applications, uniformly deep ablation is produced in the long axis of the slit and the surface curvature is reduced only in the meridian in which the slit widens. An ablatable mask is a plate of PMMA placed in the path of the laser beam to shield the cornea. The thinner areas of the mask are ablated first and therefore allow deeper ablation of the corresponding area of the cornea.

Excimer laser correction of hypermetropia is difficult and not as widely applied as to myopia. More tissue must be ablated peripherally than centrally to make the cornea steeper. This may be achieved by the use of an appropriate ablatable mask.

Laser intrastromal keratomileusis (LASIK)

A mechanical microkeratome is used to dissect through the superficial corneal stroma and fashion a lamellar circular flap of uniform thickness. The dissection is not completed and the flap remains attached at one point, which acts as a hinge so that the flap may be lifted and replaced in the same orientation. The bared corneal stroma is reshaped using an excimer laser and the hinged flap is replaced – hence the sobriquet 'flap and zap'. If under correction or regression of the refractive error occurs, the flap can be lifted to apply further treatment. Compared with PRK there appears to be little subepithelial scarring and myopic regression, earlier stabilisation of the refraction, and a superior predictability in the treatment of very high myopia.

Radial keratotomy (RK)

Radial keratotomy is a method of irreversibly flattening the central corneal curvature to reduce its refractive power and correct myopia. Partial thickness radial incisions are placed symmetrically in the mid-peripheral and peripheral cornea, sparing the central zone (Fig. 17.1). This weakens the cornea sufficiently to allow the intraocular pressure to cause the wounds to gape and the mid-peripheral and peripheral cornea to bulge. The adult cornea does not stretch and so this change in conformation causes flattening of the central cornea.

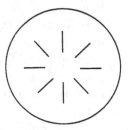

Fig. 17.1   Radial keratotomy to correct myopia.

The corneal thickness is first measured precisely using an ultrasound pachymeter (cf pp. 207–209). The depth of the incisions should be 80–90% of the corneal thickness to have any effect. A diamond knife is used which has a micrometer to allow the distance the blade projects beyond the foot-plates to be set. The footplates rest on the cornea and prevent the blade from incising too deeply.

A greater effect is achieved by longer or deeper incisions, more incisions or a smaller central zone. A surgical algorithm is used to determine these details for each eye. The diameter of the central zone should be between 3 and 5 mm; any less will risk glare from the incisions and any more will have little effect on refraction. Comparable results are obtained using either four or eight incisions. Four allows the opportunity to make further incisions to treat under-correction, and this strategy may result in fewer patients being overcorrected.

Best results are obtained for myopes of less than –5.00 D in whom more than three-quarters end up within 1.00 D of emmetropia. The refraction is stable after six months in most patients, but in a quarter or more a hypermetropic shift of up to 1.00 D continues over the next few years. Patients requiring additional optical correction after RK may be difficult or impossible to fit with contact lenses because of the altered shape of the cornea.

Surgical correction of astigmatism

Astigmatism may originate in the cornea or the lens; it may be physiological or follow surgery or other trauma. Spectacles do not adequately correct irregular astigmatism or high degrees of regular astigmatism (cf. Chapter 10, p. 115). These are best corrected by rigid contact lenses or surgery. The surgical correction of astigmatism is often unpredictable, and success is sometimes measured by the post-operative tolerance of spectacles or contact lenses to correct the residual refractive error rather than by its complete elimination.

Post-keratoplasty astigmatism (see below) is frequently irregular and its correction presents a challenge: the meridia of maximum and minimum curvature may not be at right angles to each other. Furthermore, zones of maximum and minimum curvature may be randomly distributed around the circumference of the corneal graft. Continuous sutures, interrupted sutures, a combination of both or double continuous sutures all have potential advantages in reducing graft astigmatism. Keratoscopy allows a certain amount of adjustment to be carried out during surgery to leave the cornea roughly spherical. Later adjustment may be made by redistributing tension along a continuous suture or by selectively removing interrupted sutures in the steeper meridia. Such manipulations are more exact if guided by computerised analysis of the corneal topography. When astigmatism is not amenable to further suture manipulation, other surgical or laser techniques outlined below may be used.

Relaxing incisions – transverse and arcuate keratotomy

The incision of the cornea causes it to bulge at that site. This reduces the surface curvature of the central cornea in the meridian in which the incision is made and induces increased curvature in the meridian at 90° to it (Fig. 17.2).

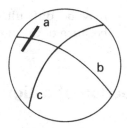

Fig. 17.2 A corneal incision (a) causes flattening of surface curvature in the same meridian as the incision (c) and steepening of the meridian 90° away (b).

This is often used after corneal grafting and also to control astigmatism in healthy corneas during cataract surgery. For example, the placement of the incision for small incision cataract surgery can be used to reduce pre-existing corneal astigmatism if the incision is made in the steepest meridian of the cornea.

Astigmatism persisting after all corneal graft sutures have been removed may be corrected by incising the graft–host junction over 60–90° where it is crossed by the meridian of steepest corneal curvature. An improvement of this technique is to place the incisions wholly within the graft. This conserves the wound and has a more predictable effect. The incisions are made tangential or curvilinear to the central zone (Fig. 17.3). An arcuate incision has the theoretical advantage that it is cut in cornea of uniform thickness and it is also concentric with the visual axis and likely to produce a more regular effect. Linear incisions pass through cornea of varying thickness, and parts of the incision are closer to the visual axis than

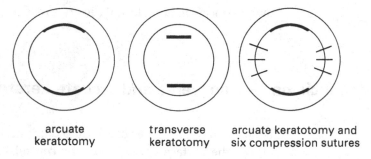

arcuate
keratotomy

transverse
keratotomy

arcuate keratotomy and
six compression sutures

Fig. 17.3 Configurations for corneal incisions to reduce astigmatism, alone (left, middle) or in combination with radial sutures (right).

others. Longer incisions or incisions closer to the visual axis have a greater effect. Nomograms are available which relate the astigmatic correction from different combinations of clear zone diameter, incision arc and the number of incisions.

Compressive techniques – wedge resection

High degrees (more than 10.0 D) of astigmatism after penetrating keratoplasty may be corrected by removing a deep arcuate wedge measuring 60–90° from the graft–host junction in the flattest meridian. The effect is the reverse of a relaxing keratotomy. The wound is sutured with non-absorbable mersilene to shorten the cornea and steepen the curvature in that meridian.

Compression sutures

A tight suture placed across the graft–host junction in the flattest meridian increases the curvature of the cornea and reduces astigmatism (Fig. 17.4). The topography will change if the sutures are removed for overcorrection or if they degenerate.

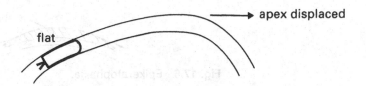

apex displaced

flat

Fig. 17.4 A tight corneal suture flattens the cornea adjacent to it and displaces the corneal apex away from it, causing the cornea to bulge away.

Relaxing incisions may be combined with compression sutures placed 90° away from them to reduce large degrees of corneal astigmatism (Fig. 17.3).

Other refractive surgery techniques

Intrastromal corneal ring (ICR)

This procedure entails placing a PMMA split ring (Fig. 17.5) into a tunnel within the mid-peripheral corneal stroma concentric with the limbus. It causes flattening of the central corneal curvature to treat myopia up to –4.00 D. The central zone of the cornea is untouched. The procedure is reversed by removal of the ring.

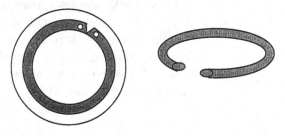

Fig. 17.5   Intrastromal corneal ring.

Epikeratophakia

This uncommon surgical technique creates a new corneal surface with a different surface curvature by attaching a lenticule of pre-shaped donor corneal stroma to the surface of the host cornea (Fig. 17.6). The eye is not entered and the procedure is easily reversed by removal of the lenticule.

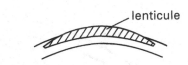

lenticule

Fig. 17.6   Epikeratophakia.

High degrees of hypermetropia and myopia may be corrected by lenticules of different spherical power. The posterior surface of the lenticule matches the surface contour of the host cornea. Care must be taken to ensure that surgery does not alter the shape of the recipient cornea which would induce unwanted refractive error. The procedure is no longer used to correct myopia because the refractive outcome was so variable and most cases of aphakia are now corrected by a secondary intraocular lens. However, epikeratophakia may still be useful in cases of aphakia or cataract where there is contact lens intolerance or an intraocular lens is contraindicated.

Epikeratophakia is most commonly employed to correct keratoconus but the surgical technique used is quite different from that used for the correction of myopia or hypermetropia. To correct keratoconus, a lenticule of uniform thickness is sutured tightly on to the conical host cornea in order to compress it and return it to a more normal contour, thereby neutralising myopia.

Keratomileusis and keratophakia

Keratomileusis is the use of a microkeratome to remove a lamella of anterior corneal stroma which is then shaped on a cryolathe before being replaced. High degrees of myopia but not of hypermetropia can be corrected in this way.

Keratophakia was developed as a modification of keratomileusis in order to correct aphakia. A keratome is used to lift a lamella of anterior stroma and this is replaced over a shaped lenticule of donor corneal stroma to produce a new corneal surface contour (Fig. 17.7). Neither technique has been widely adopted because they are technically difficult and the refractive outcome is often unpredictable.

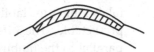

Fig. 17.7 Keratophakia.

Thermokeratoplasty

This procedure is largely experimental. A focal low temperature burn induces contraction of collagen in the peripheral cornea and increases the corneal curvature in the same meridian. The Holmium:YAG laser has superseded the use of cautery.

Clear lens extraction

The predictability and safety of small incision cataract surgery has provided the impetus for the removal of non-cataractous lenses with the insertion of an intraocular lens to correct any spherical refractive error. This has been advocated for high myopia and for hypermetropes with presbyopia.

Phakic intraocular lenses

Intraocular lenses have also been placed in the anterior or posterior chambers of phakic eyes to correct refractive errors. It is claimed that they correct higher refractive errors more predictably than corneal procedures whilst conserving accommodation. The long-term effects of these lenses on the corneal endothelium, crystalline lens and irido-corneal angle are not known.

Corneal incisions

Corneal incisions which are longer, deeper or closer to the visual axis have the greatest effect on the central corneal curvature. Those which are smaller and further from the visual axis are more astigmatically neutral. Longer corneal incisions are more unstable and therefore slower to heal. Corneal healing is also significantly slower in the old than the young. Delayed healing means that any refractive error takes longer to stabilise and the effect of the surgery is less predictable. The effects of incisions which are radial or parallel to the limbus have been discussed above (p. 248).

The large corneal incision used for intracapsular and extracapsular cataract surgery must be closed by sutures. The wound edges are apposed by either interrupted or continuous sutures. In the case of interrupted sutures, a tight radial suture induces corneal astigmatism by increasing the corneal curvature in that meridian. The suture may need to be removed when the wound has healed. A suture which is looser than others reduces the corneal curvature in that meridian. A continuous suture may cause less astigmatism by distributing the tension more evenly along the wound. Degradation of suture material reduces its tensile strength and may cause a gradual change in refractive error for as long as a year following surgery.

The small self-sealing incision used in phacoemulsification cataract surgery tends to flatten the cornea in the same meridian post-operatively. The temporal limbus is further from the visual axis, and incisions here therefore tend to be more astigmatically neutral than those located elsewhere. One may use surgically induced astigmatism to neutralise pre-operative corneal astigmatism by placing the incision in the steeper axis. Alternatively, some surgeons always use a temporal incision but overcome corneal astigmatism by placing astigmatic keratotomies in the steeper axis.

Penetrating keratoplasty (PK)

The refractive outcome of penetrating keratoplasty is determined in part by the dimensions of the donor tissue. A graft whose diameter exceeds that of the tissue removed from the host is more likely to result in myopia. Corneas from paediatric donors have greater surface curvature and refractive power and may be used in aphakic eyes requiring penetrating keratoplasty.

Vitreo-retinal surgery

The repair of a retinal detachment frequently requires the attachment of a silicone buckle to the sclera in order to indent the wall of the eye. This will cause the axial length of the eye to increase and induce myopia, especially if the buckle encircles the eye (Fig. 17.8). Buckles are also likely to cause astigmatism if they compress the eye asymmetrically, for example radial or partial circumferential buckles. This effect is reversed after the buckle is removed.

Silicone oil in the posterior segment of the eye has a higher refractive index than the crystalline lens and changes the posterior surface of the lens from a converging to a diverging interface. This induces a hypermetropic shift in refraction of the order of +5.00 to +7.00 D. In an aphakic eye, the curved anterior surface and higher refractive index of

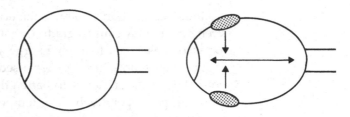

Fig. 17.8 An encircling scleral buckle constricts the globe and increases the axial length.

silicone oil compared with the crystalline lens is more strongly converging and therefore produces a myopic shift. The hypermetropia which normally results from aphakia will therefore be of the order of only +4.00 to +6.00 D.

Gas in the posterior segment of a phakic eye greatly increases the refractive power of the posterior surface of the lens and causes a large myopic shift; this may allow indirect ophthalmoscopy without the use of a condensing lens. Gas filling an aphakic eye makes the posterior corneal surface highly diverging and almost neutralises the refractive power of the cornea to allow an unaided view of the fundus.

Appendix I

Mathematical definitions

1. Sine, Cosine and Tangent.

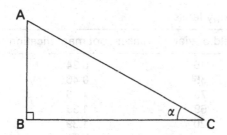

$$\text{Sine } \alpha = \frac{AB}{AC}$$

$$\text{Cosine } \alpha = \frac{BC}{AC}$$

$$\text{Tan } \alpha = \frac{AB}{BC}$$

2. Angles formed by parallel lines

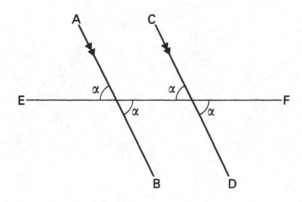

The angles α formed by parallel lines AB and CD intersecting line EF are all equal.

Appendix II

Specifications of various indirect ophthalmoscopy lenses.

Lens	Angular magnification	Field of view	Laser spot magnification
20D	2.97	46°	0.34
28D	2.16	55°	0.46
78D	0.87	73°	1.15
90D	0.72	69°	1.39
Superfield	0.72	120°	1.39

Larger diameter lenses give a larger field of view.

Index